Date: 7/9/13

616.85841 ASH
Ashley, Larry L.
The truth about gambling /

THE TRUTH ABOUT GAMBLING

THE TRUTH ABOUT GAMBLING

Robert N. Golden, M.D.
University of Wisconsin-Madison
General Editor

Fred L. Peterson, Ph.D.
University of Texas-Austin
General Editor

Larry L. Ashley, Ed.S., LCADC, CPGC,
Meghan E. Pierce, and Fred L. Peterson, Ph.D.
Principal Authors

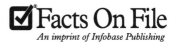
Facts On File
An imprint of Infobase Publishing

The Truth About Gambling

Facts On File, Inc.
An imprint of Infobase Publishing
132 West 31st Street
New York NY 10001

Library of Congress Cataloging-in-Publication Data

Ashley, Larry L.
  The truth about gambling / Robert N. Golden, general editor, Fred L. Peterson, general editor ; Larry L. Ashley, Meghan E. Pierce, and Fred L. Peterson, principal authors.
      p. cm.
  Includes bibliographical references and index.
  ISBN-13: 978-0-8160-7638-3 (hardcover : alk. paper)
  ISBN-10: 0-8160-7638-3 (hardcover : alk. paper) 1. Compulsive gambling. 2. Compulsive —Psychological aspects. 3. Gambling. 4. Gambling—Psychological aspects. I. Pierce, Meghan E. II. Peterson, Fred L. III. Golden, Robert N. IV. Title.
  RC569.5.G35A84 2011
  616.85'841—dc22   2010045440

Text design by David Strelecky
Composition by Kerry Casey
Cover printed by Yurchak Printing, Inc., Landisville, Pa.
Book printed and bound by Yurchak Printing, Inc., Landisville, Pa.
Date printed: July 2011
Printed in the United States of America

10 9 8 7 6 5 4 3 2 1

This book is printed on acid-free paper.

CONTENTS

LIST OF ILLUSTRATIONS

PREFACE

The Truth About series—updated and expanded to include 20 volumes—
seeks to identify the most pressing health issues and social challenges
confronting our nation's youth. Adolescence is the period between the
onset of puberty and the attainment of adult roles and responsibilities.
Adolescence is also a time of storm, stress, and risk-taking for many
young people. During adolescence, a person's health is influenced by
biological, psychological, and social factors, all of which interact with
one's environment—family, peers, school, and community. It is a time
when teenagers experience profound changes.

With the latest available statistics and new insights that have
emerged from ongoing research, the Truth About series seeks to help
young people build a foundation of information as they face some
of the challenges that will affect their health and well-being. These
challenges include high-risk behaviors, such as alcohol, tobacco, and
other drug use; sexual behaviors that can lead to adolescent pregnancy and sexually transmitted diseases (STDs), such as HIV/AIDS;
mental health concerns, such as depression and suicide; learning disorders and disabilities, which are often associated with school failures
and school drop-outs; serious family problems, including domestic
violence and abuse; and lifestyle factors, which increase adolescents'
risk for noncommunicable diseases, such as diabetes and cardiovas-
cular disease, among others.

Broader underlying factors also influence adolescent health. These
include socioeconomic circumstances, such as poverty, available
health care, and the political and social situations in which young
people live. Although these factors can negatively affect adolescent

health and well-being, as well as school performance, many of these negative health outcomes are preventable with the proper knowledge and information.

With prevention in mind, the writers and editors of each topical volume in the Truth About series have tried to provide cutting-edge information that is supported by research and scientific evidence. Vital facts are presented that inform youth about the challenges experienced during adolescence, while special features seek to dispel common myths and misconceptions. Some of the main topics explored include abuse, alcohol, death and dying, divorce, drugs, eating disorders, family life, fear and depression, rape, sexual behavior and unplanned pregnancy, smoking, and violence. All volumes discuss risk-taking behaviors and their consequences, healthy choices, prevention, available treatments, and where to get help.

In this new edition of the series, we also have added eight new titles in areas of increasing significance to today's youth. ADHD, or attention-deficit/hyperactivity disorder, and learning disorders are diagnosed with increasing frequency, and many students have observed or know of classmates receiving treatment for these conditions, even if they have not themselves received this diagnosis. Gambling is gaining currency in our culture, as casinos open and expand in many parts of the country, and the Internet offers easy access for this addictive behavior. Another consequence of our increasingly "online" society, unfortunately, is the presence of online predators. Environmental hazards represent yet another danger, and it is important to provide unbiased information about this topic to our youth. Suicide, which for many years has been a "silent epidemic," is now gaining recognition as a major public health problem throughout the life span, including the teenage and young adult years. We now also offer an overview of illness and disease in a volume that includes the major conditions of particular interest and concern to youth. In addition to illness, however, it is essential to emphasize health and its promotion, and this is especially apparent in the volumes on physical fitness and stress management.

It is our intent that each book serve as an accessible, authoritative resource that young people can turn for accurate and meaningful answers to their specific questions. The series can help them research particular problems and provide an up-to-date evidence base. It is also designed with parents, teachers, and counselors in mind so that they have a reliable resource that they can share with youth who seek their guidance.

Finally, we have tried to provide unbiased facts rather than subjective opinions. Our goal is to help elevate the health of the public with an emphasis on its most precious component—our youth. As young people face the challenges of an increasingly complex world, we as educators want them to be armed with the most powerful weapon available—knowledge.

Robert N. Golden, M.D.
Fred L. Peterson, Ph.D.
General Editors

HOW TO USE THIS BOOK

NOTE TO STUDENTS

Knowledge is power. By possessing knowledge you have the ability to make decisions, ask follow-up questions, or know where to go to obtain more information. In the world of health that *is* power! That is the purpose of this book—to provide you with the power you need to obtain unbiased, accurate information and *The Truth About Gambling.*

Topics in each volume of The Truth About series are arranged in alphabetical order, from A to Z. Each of these entries defines its topic and explains in detail the particular issue. At the end of most entries are cross-references to related topics. A list of all topics by letter can be found in the table of contents or at the back of the book in the index.

How have these books been compiled? First, the publisher worked with me to identify some of the country's leading authorities on key issues in health education. These individuals were asked to identify some of the major concerns that young people have about such topics. The writers read the literature, spoke with health experts, and incorporated their own life and professional experiences to pull together the most up-to-date information on health issues, particularly those of interest to adolescents and of concern in Healthy People 2010.

Throughout the alphabetical entries, the reader will find sidebars that separate Fact from Fiction. There are Question-and-Answer boxes that attempt to address the most common questions that youths ask about sensitive topics. In addition, readers will find a special feature called "Teens Speak"—case studies of teens with personal stories related to the topic in hand.

This may be one of the most important books you will ever read. Please share it with your friends, families, teachers, and classmates. Remember, you possess the power to control your future. One way to affect your course is through the acquisition of knowledge. Good luck and keep healthy.

NOTE TO LIBRARIANS

This book, along with the rest of The Truth About series, serves as a wonderful resource for young researchers. It contains a variety of facts, case studies, and further readings that the reader can use to help answer questions, formulate new questions, or determine where to go to find more information. Even though the topics may be considered delicate by some, do not be afraid to ask patrons if they have questions. Feel free to direct them to the appropriate sources, but do not press them if you encounter reluctance. The best we can do as educators is to let young people know that we are there when they need us.

ACKNOWLEDGMENTS

I would like to especially acknowledge my coauthor Meghan Pierce, who is also my Harrah's Graduate Assistant in Problem Gambling Counseling. In addition to her excellent writing, Meghan oversaw the following individuals who helped gather data that was invaluable to this book: Karmen Boelke, Erika Flores, Micheala Novak, Becky Homer, Viridiana Linares-Vital, Charles Mrozak, and Shawna Watts. In addition, a very special thanks goes to Dr. Kenneth Winters, director of the Center for Adolescent Substance Abuse Research at the University of Minnesota, and to Keith Whyte, executive director of the National Council on Problem Gambling.

ADOLESCENT GAMBLING: RISKING THE FUTURE

Placing a "friendly" bet, or **wager,** with a buddy on which sports team will win a championship is a commonplace activity not only for adults, but, despite its illegal nature, for adolescents. In gambling, people choose **risk** over a certain outcome; they enjoy the potential thrill of success as well as the uncertainty that is provided by betting on some event.

Gambling is an increasingly popular leisure activity in the United States, and it has become a popular pursuit among adolescents. In fact, according to the *Journal of Gambling Studies* in a 2010 article, "between 60 and 99% of young people aged 12–20 years have gambled," and the number is on the rise. Most youth gamble for entertainment, even though they are **underage.** However, about one in four teens appear to be motivated to gamble just to beat an opponent, for the thrill of a risky competition, and to make money, all of which are reasons associated with potential harm for young people.

UNDERAGE GAMBLING

Although the law differs from state to state, gambling in most states is illegal for those under 21. In 11 states and in Washington, D.C., it is illegal for those under 18. However, finding adults to help underage teens break the law is not difficult for the problem gambler. Also, just as they do to engage in underage drinking, some teens will obtain fake ID's in order to gamble in a casino.

1

The legal gambling age at most online sites is generally 18. Because many online gambling "casinos" are based outside of the United States, they are not subject to U.S. rules and regulations. Also, if an adolescent has access to a legitimate credit card, enforcement of the law is almost impossible. In fact, according to the 2008 National Annenberg Survey of Youth, "more than 300,000 youth in the study age range (14–22) gamble for money at least once a week on the Internet, and over 700,000 [youth] do so at least once a month." Despite the passage in 2006 of the Unlawful Internet Gambling Enforcement Act (UIGEA), also according to the Annenberg study, young people "are still risking their financial futures on [Internet] poker."

THE TRUTH ABOUT PROBLEM GAMBLING

This volume takes a comprehensive look at the role of gambling in society—examining the biological, psychological, social, and environmental factors that influence the decision of adolescents to gamble. Articles on addiction, family life, peer pressure, public health issues, risk taking, and more explore how gambling is a pervasive and potentially **addictive** behavior that can affect all aspects of one's life. Although the legal gambling age differs from state to state, all gambling is illegal under 18 years of age. However, there are abundant opportunities and places for teens to gamble, including

- poker tournaments in residence halls, fraternities, and student unions
- school- and student organization–sponsored events
- tournaments at local bars or clubs
- online contests
- Internet gambling
- sports betting
- TV shows
- community events
- gatherings of family and friends
- dormitory competitions
- raffles
- casinos
- riverboats

- lotteries
- pull tabs
- video games

According to therapists, counselors, and researchers, there are different levels of gambling which range on a continuum from:

No gambling → Social gambling → At-risk gambling →
Compulsive gambling → Problem gambling →
Pathological gambling → Habitual gambling

Among young people on the continuum, according to a June 2010 report in the *Journal of Gambling Studies,* the prevalence rate ranges between 0.9 and 23.5 percent for problem gambling. Although the wide range is the result of different populations (in America, Canada, and Australia) being measured in multiple studies using a range of assessment tools, the numbers are significant. Also, when looking just at adolescent pathological gamblers, toward the end of the continuum, recent North American studies indicate that between 4.4 and 7.4 percent of young people have a serious gambling problem.

ADDICTIVE BEHAVIOR

Gambling is prevalent among adolescents from as early as the elementary school years, and problem gambling is emerging as a risk-taking behavior that is not only destructive to youth but also a public health issue. Studies show that gambling can cause personal, emotional, and financial difficulties for those involved, which in turn places a significant burden on society. Gambling behavior in adolescents also has been linked to other risk-taking behaviors, such as drug and alcohol abuse. Unfortunately, while there are reports of **pathological** gambling beginning as early as age nine or 10, the problem often goes unnoticed due to a lack of observable signs.

Gambling can be a powerful form of addiction, and research suggests that young people may have more trouble controlling their gambling behavior than adults. Teens have a greater propensity for a behavioral addiction such as gambling for several reasons: immature brain development of their pre-frontal cortex (decision-making center); teen impulsivity; and the production of brain chemicals (**neurotransmitters**) that provide the sense of pleasure, excitement, and psychological arousal. In fact, rates of problem gambling among youth are considerably higher than the rates for adult problem gambling.

Not only are teenagers at greater risk of experiencing problems associated with gambling behavior, but those who gamble as adolescents are at greater risk of becoming problem gamblers and experiencing gambling-related difficulties as adults.

Trends among adolescent gamblers

Because frequent gambling in adolescence may develop into problem gambling in adulthood, understanding the prevalence and risk factors for adolescent problem gambling is an important issue that ultimately may help to reduce the social and public health problems associated with problem gambling. In fact, according to recent reports by Dr. Jeffrey L. Derevensky, a leading scholar in Youth Gambling Behavior at the International Centre for Youth Gambling Problems and High Risk Behaviors at McGill University in Montreal, Canada, the majority of adult problem gamblers had a gambling problem prior to age 20, with some starting as young as eight years old.

In March 2010, Dr. Derevensky reported the following trends among adolescents who gamble:

- Adolescent pathological gamblers are greater risk-takers.
- Adolescent prevalence rates of problem gambling are two to four times that of adults.
- Gambling has become a family activity:
  - 40–68 percent of youth gamble with family members.
  - 80–90 percent of parents report knowing their children gamble for money and do not object.
  - 77 percent of adolescents report their parents purchased lottery tickets for them.
- Adolescents with gambling problems have poor general coping skills.
- Few adolescents fear getting caught gambling.
- Adolescent problem gamblers report beginning gambling at earlier ages, approximately 10 years of age.
- There is rapid movement from social gambler to problem gambler.

Characteristics of adolescent gamblers

Dr. Derevensky also reports the following characteristics of an adolescent problem gambler:

- lower self-esteem compared with other adolescents
- higher rates of depression
- heightened risk for suicide ideation and suicide attempts
- increased delinquency and criminal behaviors
- disruption of familial relationships
- decreased academic performance
- has old friends replaced by gambling associates
- remains at increased risk for the development of an addiction or multiple addictions
- scores lower on measures of conformity, self-discipline, and resiliency in light of risk factors
- has experienced more major life events and early childhood traumas
- is more likely to have parents with a gambling problem, some other mental health issue, or a substance abuse problem

Despite these negative consequences, most adolescents view gambling as socially acceptable and less harmful than alcohol, drugs, or cigarettes. Most also believe that gambling is a relatively benign activity. As reported by Dr. Deverensky:

- 40 percent of [study] participants believe that playing cards for money is harmless even when played at least once a week.
- 37 percent believe that teens should be allowed to use video lottery terminals (VLTs).
- While 72 percent agree that gambling can be bad for you, 28 percent of the participants either disagree or are neutral in this matter.

Profile of an adolescent problem gambler
Teens who have developed into problem gamblers tend to have certain traits and/or circumstances:

- predominantly male
- significantly anxious
- have family problems and poor peer relationships
- unable to stop gambling despite repeated efforts

- have serious financial difficulties
- failures in school and/or at work
- prone to lying
- prone to stealing (from family, friends, stores, etc.)
- depressed
- ineffective at coping and problem solving
- confused and conflicted about whether they really want to stop gambling

HEALTHY RISKS

Finally, readers will find that *The Truth About Gambling* is a comprehensive overview of problem gambling and of the sometimes risky and illegal behavior of gambling by adolescents. Underage gambling is an unhealthy risk that can lead to many personal and physical health problems as well as other destructive behaviors. Although there are numerous biological, psychological, social, and environmental factors that contribute to a person's gambling during adolescence, making it a potential danger, the hope of the authors and other experts is that young people instead will elect risk-taking challenges that are fun and safe, that fulfill the need for healthy and legal thrill seeking. Unhealthy risks—such as using alcohol, tobacco, and other drugs; eating disorders; unprotected sexual activity; involvement in violent neighborhood gangs; self-injury; suicide; shoplifting; and problem gambling—should be avoided.

There are many sensational activities that are considered healthy risks, such as invigorating physical activity, horseback riding, skating, rock climbing, white-water rafting, raising animals, volunteering for community service, helping the needy in one's community, competing for a scholarship, going to college to prepare for a desired career, learning a new skill or creative art, and more. These activities enrich a person's life. Adolescence is an opportunity to pursue one's dreams and experience the satisfaction of taking risks that are healthy and legal.

RISKY BUSINESS SELF-TEST

The following test is designed to let you find out more about your own risk of becoming a problem gambler or to identify if you are now. Record your answers on a separate sheet of paper. For each question, answer "yes" for those behaviors that describe your actions and "no" for those that do not.

___Do you find yourself thinking about gambling activities at odd times of the day and/or planning the next time you will play?

___Do you find the need to spend more and more money on gambling activities?

___Do you owe money to more and more people?

___Do you become restless, tense, fed up, or bad-tempered when trying to cut down or stop gambling?

___Do you ever gamble as a way of escaping from problems?

___After losing money on gambling activities, do you (more than half the time) play again another day and try to win back the money you lost?

___Do you lie to your family and friends to hide how much you gamble?

___Do you talk frequently and/or boast about gambling?

___In the past year, have you spent your school lunch money, or money for bus or train fares, on gambling activities?

___In the past year, have you secretly taken money from someone you live with to gamble?

___In the past year, have you stolen money from outside the family, or shoplifted, to gamble?

___Have you fallen out with members of your family or with close friends because of your gambling behavior?

___In the past year, have you missed school (five times or more) to participate in gambling experiences?

___In the past year, have you gone to someone for help with a serious money worry caused by participation in gambling activities?

If you answered *yes* to four or more of the questions in the above self-test, you may have a gambling problem. If you think you have a problem, talk to a trusted adult—a parent, a school counselor, a clergy member—and seek professional assistance. Treatment is available.

A-TO-Z ENTRIES

■ ADDICTION AND GAMBLING

The inability to stop a behavior despite significant negative physical and psychological effects and **pathological** gambling. Like gambling, alcohol and drug use and other **addictive** behaviors are generally viewed as occurring along a continuum. At any particular time, individuals may fall into any one of the following five levels of **chemical** or behavioral involvement: abstainers, social users, substance abusers, **addicts** who are physically dependent (but not psychologically dependent), and addicts who are both physically and psychologically dependent.

The term *addiction* (derived from the Latin *addicere,* meaning "to adore or surrender oneself to a master") was initially applied to the disorder known as **alcoholism.** However, over time, addiction has been used to describe other behaviors of **dependency,** such as excessive or dependent drug use, sex, work, gambling, buying, eating, and Internet use.

THE DEVELOPMENT OF ADDICTION

Addiction is a complex phenomenon comprised of a complicated set of factors, including biological, psychological, and sociological determinants. As a result of the large number of variables related to the onset of addiction, ideas about and explanations for addiction abound.

The multiple numbers of addiction theories and models make it clear that no one single model or theory can be used to explain why or how addictions develop. In fact, to date, there is no universally accepted definition of addiction. Rather, a variety of theories or models have been presented over time. While not all-inclusive, the following list represents some of the more predominant perspectives from which addiction, including excessive gambling, has been and continues to be described, explained, and treated.

Moral model

Dating back to the 1850s, this model defines an addict as weak in character. Its foundation lies on the idea that individuals have free choice and, as a result, are responsible for their behaviors. This approach has significantly influenced both public policy and the judicial system in America.

Medical/disease model

Proposed by Dr. Benjamin Rush in the early 1800s, this model, formally accepted as the definition of addiction by the American Medical

Association (AMA) in 1945, identifies addiction as a physical disease, rather than as a **mental disorder** or a moral failing. According to the AMA, the disease may go into **remission,** but there is no known cure.

Genetic model
Over the past 20 years, researchers have identified in some individuals a **genetic** predisposition to alcohol, tobacco, and other often abused substances. In other words, according to this model, addiction is heritable, meaning it can be inherited.

Social-learning model
This model suggests that individuals are likely to repeat the actions they observe in others. Therefore, according to this theory, individuals become addicts because they model the behaviors they see in their parents, siblings, and peers.

Cognitive-behavior model
Based on the assumption that thinking underlies all behavior, this model assumes that illogical or irrational thinking underlies the development of addiction.

Self-medication model
This view originated in the 1960s among psychoanalysts. It assumes that individuals self-medicate in order to cope with life's problems. In other words, the theory suggests that a person in emotional pain will self-medicate in order to find relief.

Impulse-control disorder model
From this perspective, addiction occurs because either **neurobiological** or genetic deficiencies make an individual unable to control or regulate impulsive behavior. Under certain conditions, these individuals will put themselves at risk and find temporary relief with self-destructive behaviors such as kleptomania, pyromania, drug **abuse,** and gambling.

Biomedical model
This theory of addiction draws from both the biological and behavioral sciences. Essentially, it suggests that gambling or using alcohol or other drugs repeatedly over time changes both the structure and

the function of the brain. These changes can persist long after an individual stops using the substance(s) or ceases the behavior(s). In other words, once the addiction impacts the brain, an individual is driven to support the demands made by the brain in order to prevent becoming ill from the symptoms of withdrawal.

Bio-psycho-social model

Developed in the 1980s, this model asserts that an individual's vulnerability for developing an addiction is affected by the complex interaction among one's physical status (function of the body); one's psychological state (how one views and perceives the world); and one's social dynamics (how and with whom one interacts).

Public health model

In 1989, the Institute of Medicine (IOM) defined addiction from a public health perspective. The organization identified three causative factors: agents (such as psychoactive drugs); hosts (individuals who differ in their genetic, physiological, behavioral, and sociocultural susceptibility to various forms of chemicals); and environment (the availability and accessibility of the agents).

THE FIVE CHARACTERISTICS OF ADDICTION

Regardless of how an addiction is manifested—through chemical use (for example, alcohol or cocaine) or behaviors (such as cybersex or compulsive gambling)—addictions generally share these five characteristics:

1. compulsive use: This concept refers to reinforcement, craving, and habit. Reinforcement occurs when the substance or behavior is first engaged. Being rewarded with pleasure and/or relief from pain and stress reinforce the user. Craving means that the body and brain send intense signals that the drug or behavior is needed. Habit results from deeply ingrained patterns in the memory of the nervous system.

2. loss of control: Typically, addicts cannot predict or determine how much of a drug or behavior they will use or when they will use a drug or engage in a harmful behavior. However, once they begin, they cannot stop. This may be due in part to impairment of the brain and

memory. This same loss of control that applies to drug abuse also applies to behavioral addictions such as compulsive gambling or sexual activity.

3. continued use despite adverse consequences: Addictions generate negative consequences. Addicts may be unaware of these consequences, or, if they are aware, they may feel that the pleasurable or pain-relieving features of the drug or the behavior outweigh the problems incurred by the behavior.

4. tolerance: When a drug is used continually, the body adapts and begins to tolerate the pharmacological effects. As a result, the user needs increasingly more of the substance or the behavior in order to achieve the desired feeling or outcome. Additionally, the **chronic** abuser must also take more drugs or engage in more harmful activity in order to avoid the physical discomfort and psychological distress that accompany withdrawal when they stop.

5. withdrawal: When drug use is stopped or behavior is ceased, the addict suffers unpleasant symptoms that are usually the opposite of those induced by the chemical or the behavior. Because the body has adapted to the drug or behavior, withdrawal (unless carefully managed and monitored by a doctor or other professional) is not only miserable, it also may be life-threatening.

BEHAVIORAL DEPENDENCIES

Many individuals have difficulty seeing pathological gambling, or many of the other behavioral dependencies, as an addiction similar to alcoholism or drug addiction. It is easy to see why. With alcohol or other drugs, an individual introduces substances into his or her body and, as a result, observable biological and chemical changes occur. When gambling, no substance enters the body. However, excessive gambling, similar to other addictive behaviors, is a multidimensional disorder or condition involving bio-psycho-social determinants. These include a physiological predisposition to the behavior, environmental stressors, social and familial influences, psychological processes, and individual personality characteristics.

Symptoms of Pathological Gambling

According the to the APA's diagnostic criteria, pathological gambling is defined as "persistent and recurrent maladaptive gambling behavior" as indicated by five or more of the following 10 symptoms:

1. preoccupation with gambling, such as reliving past gambling experiences, handicapping upcoming events, planning the next venture, or thinking of ways to get money in which to gamble

2. the need to bet increasing amounts of money in order to achieve the desired excitement

3. repeated unsuccessful efforts to control, cut back, or stop gambling

4. restlessness or irritability when attempting to cut down or stop gambling

5. using gambling as an escape from problems or to relieve feelings of helplessness, guilt, anxiety, or depression

6. "chasing" losses, or after losing money gambling, returning soon afterward with the aim of getting even

7. lying to family members, a therapist, or others to conceal the extent of the involvement with gambling

8. committing illegal acts, such as forgery, fraud, theft, or embezzlement to finance gambling

9. having jeopardized or lost a significant relationship, job, or educational or career opportunity because of gambling

10. relying on others to provide money to relieve a desperate financial situation caused by gambling

An individual who exhibits five or more of the 10 criteria found in the *Diagnostic and Statistical Manual of Mental Disorders (DSM)* is defined as a pathological gambler. Individuals who exhibit fewer than five of the *DSM* criteria are defined as problem gamblers. Neither social gambling nor professional gambling is considered a disorder.

Changes in the brain

Chemical changes in the brain occur during gambling, and these changes are similar to what happens when alcohol or other drugs are ingested. For instance, neuroscientists have shown that the central nervous system reward circuits for winning money parallel the reward mechanisms associated with the anticipation of cocaine use or the appreciation of female beauty by males. In addition, some gamblers experience blackouts while in action, and some experience withdrawal when they try to stop gambling. This growing body of research demonstrates that gambling can mimic the subjective effects of ingesting psychoactive drugs and that this experience can change important characteristics of the central nervous system.

Similarities between pathological gambling and chemical dependency include an inability to stop or control one's behavior, denial, depression, irritability, and mood swings. Additionally, pathological gambling and chemical dependency are **progressive disorders** that share similar phases, including "chasing" the first win or the first high, experiencing blackouts, and using the object of the addiction in order to escape pain. Both pathological gamblers and individuals addicted to alcohol or drugs are preoccupied with their addiction, experience low self-esteem, and seek immediate gratification.

In 1980, the American Psychiatric Association (APA) officially recognized pathological gambling as a mental disorder and, for the first time, included it in its diagnostic manual, the *Diagnostic and Statistical Manual of Mental Disorders (DSM)*. In the manual, the APA characterizes pathological gambling as a "disorder of Impulse Control." The APA calls the disorder "extremely incapacitating" because those who experience it run the risk of incurring a myriad of consequences including, but not limited to, financial ruin, an assortment of mental and physical health disorders, job loss, and family relationships that have been destroyed by catastrophic events.

Gambling can be a powerful form of addiction for many individuals, even adolescents. In fact, research conducted by Henry Lesieur, Ph.D., Durand Jacobs, Ph.D., and others indicates that adolescents are about three times more likely than adults to become problem gamblers. Still, although pathological gambling is a chronic and progressive illness, it can be diagnosed and treated.

See also: Adolescents and Gambling; Alcohol, Drugs, and Gambling; Social Gambling

FURTHER READING
Ruschmann, Paul. *Legalized Gambling.* New York: Chelsea House, 2008.

ADOLESCENTS AND GAMBLING

The attraction of young people to risk taking through gaming, which often results in negative outcomes. **Adolescence** is sometimes characterized in two very different ways. The first defines it as a period of fun-filled excitement, growth, and experimentation, a launch pad into a progressive and productive young adulthood. The second definition characterizes adolescence as a period of inner conflict and family discord, a time of turmoil, which has the potential to lead to dysfunction, apathy, and alienation. Arguably, for most, adolescence is composed of a combination of both, a time filled with joys and challenges.

Undoubtedly, opportunities abound during this period. However, in order to capitalize on early opportunities, it often becomes necessary to take risks. In other words, opportunities and risk taking seem to go hand-in-hand. However, risk taking tends to make individuals vulnerable not only to uncertainty, but also to both positive and negative outcomes.

For many adults, including parents and teachers, it seems obvious that adolescents enjoy taking risks. In fact, engaging in one or more high-risk behaviors is often viewed as a normal expectation during the adolescent years. Over time, psychologists and other experts have offered a number of explanations or theories to explain the apparent link between the adolescent life stage and risk taking.

REASONS FOR RISK TAKING

The following list is a summary of selected theories that seek to explain adolescents' apparent attraction to risky activities:

- Rebellion—Adolescents take risks to rebel against adult authority.
- Problem Behavior Theory—Adolescents who engage in risk taking take multiple risks and do so as a form of expressing their unconventionality.

- Sensation Seeking—A subset of adolescents possess a biological predisposition to engage in activities associated with heightened physiological arousal.

- Invulnerability—Adolescents engage in risk-taking behavior because they see themselves as invulnerable to the potential risks associated with their actions.

- Conscious Decision—Adolescents consciously decide to take risks because they perceive personal benefits from doing so.

- Immaturity and Present Orientation—Adolescents take risks because they are not yet mature enough to see the potential risks associated with the actions and because they tend to live in the present moment, making it difficult for them to consider future consequences.

The above list is not all-inclusive. However, regardless of which risk-taking explanation one applies, risky behavior holds some benefits for adolescents, such as pleasure, status, and, perhaps, increased income. On the other hand, risky behavior also has the potential to generate negative outcomes, such as peer and family conflict, failing grades, health problems, and even, in extreme cases, the loss of one's life.

EVERYONE TAKES RISKS

Taking risks is not a behavior confined to adolescents. It is, in fact, part of human nature to take risks. Throughout the course of our life span, human beings take any number of risks in many areas of our lives. For example, people take risks when beginning new relationships or ending old ones, when changing jobs, or when changing our interests or goals.

Therefore, it should not be surprising that gambling, sometimes referred to as gaming, appeals to many people. At its simplest, gambling is only another stylized form of risk taking. Defined as the practice of playing games of chance or betting with the hope of winning money or something of value, gambling always involves risk and uncertainty.

In some seemingly harmless forms and venues, gambling is popular and socially acceptable. Schools, for example, often sponsor the sale of raffle tickets as fund-raisers; churches sponsor bingo games where winners receive cash prizes or gifts; charities sell 50–50 tickets where

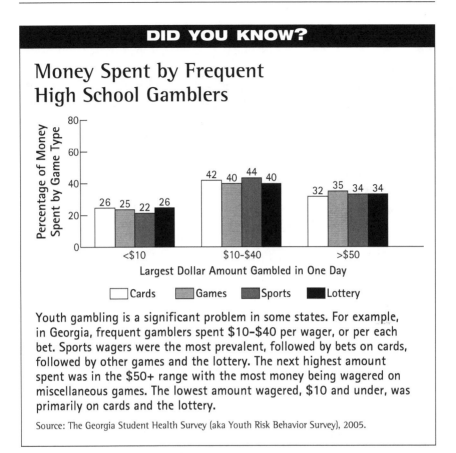

DID YOU KNOW?

Money Spent by Frequent High School Gamblers

Youth gambling is a significant problem in some states. For example, in Georgia, frequent gamblers spent $10–$40 per wager, or per each bet. Sports wagers were the most prevalent, followed by bets on cards, followed by other games and the lottery. The next highest amount spent was in the $50+ range with the most money being wagered on miscellaneous games. The lowest amount wagered, $10 and under, was primarily on cards and the lottery.

Source: The Georgia Student Health Survey (aka Youth Risk Behavior Survey), 2005.

half the proceeds are donated to the organization or cause while the winners receive the other 50 percent; and state-run lottery tickets can be purchased on nearly every street corner. These are all forms of gambling.

GAMBLING IN A YOUTH CULTURE

In the past, gambling was viewed as a primarily adult pastime characterized by thrills and risks. However, more recently, gambling activities among adolescents have increased significantly. Growing up in a society where gambling is legal and widely accepted has reduced, if not eliminated, most of the stigma that was previously associated with the activity. In fact, movies, TV shows, and increased access to gaming through the Internet have helped to embed gambling in modern youth culture.

For example, in the 1980s, it was estimated that 45 percent of teens had gambled during the past year. However, the results of multiple surveys reported in 2007 indicated that, over the past year, between 60 percent and 80 percent of all middle-school and high-school students in North America had engaged in some form of gambling for money. While most are considered to be social or recreational gamblers—those who gamble occasionally for the purpose of socialization, entertainment, and enjoyment—of the 80 percent who gamble, 10–15 percent of those teens are at risk for the development of a gambling problem. Furthermore, 3–8 percent are considered to have serious problems and are labeled problem or pathological gamblers. These rates in adolescents are significantly higher than the 1.5 percent prevalence rate of pathological gamblers in the adult population.

Fact Or Fiction?

Male teens gamble more than female teens.

The Facts: Male teens gamble more and are more likely to become involved in problem gambling than female teens. In addition, gender differences have been identified in the types of games in which males and females become involved. While females are more likely to participate in bingo, scratch cards, lotteries, and other games of chance, males are more likely to engage in games of skill, such as poker, blackjack, and sports betting. Males also appear to make larger bets and, in general, take more risks when they gamble than females.

WHY YOUTH GAMBLE

Adolescents gamble for a number of reasons. Some gamble for fun, to socialize, to win money, and to experience the thrill of the risk-win scenario. Some gamble to escape from problems at home or at school. Others gamble to avoid feeling disconnected and/or to alleviate feelings of depression and loneliness.

Gambling appears to start innocently enough: watching parents gamble, playing cards with friends for money, and participating in high school betting pools or scratch-off cards at fast-food restaurants. All these activities present ways for teens to develop firsthand experience with gambling. While most research indicates that the median age for initiating gambling is 11 to 13 years, the National Council on Problem Gambling cites other research indicating that almost half of the problem gamblers in this country began before the age of 10.

For many teens the biggest problems with gambling begin in high school. Card games and betting on sports are the most common forms of teen gambling. Poker also has become increasingly popular in association with television programs such as "Celebrity Poker" and the Poker World Series. Sports betting also has grown in popularity as a result of the American obsession with college and professional sports, and there is mounting anecdotal evidence suggesting that online gambling has increased greatly. In fact, any teen with access to both the Internet and a credit or debit card has ample opportunity to gamble. Thus, today's adolescents are one of the first generations of teens to grow up with widespread exposure to and opportunity for legal and illegal gambling.

NEGATIVE OUTCOMES

Most people who gamble are able to do so responsibly and, subsequently, do not suffer any gambling-related problems. Unfortunately, some do become addicted to various forms of gambling just as one would become addicted to drugs or alcohol. For those individuals who develop a problem or pathological gambling disorder, a myriad of consequences can and do occur.

While the negative consequences of some risky behaviors are obvious, such as the negative outcomes related to unprotected sex, for other behaviors, including teen gambling, the consequences are less immediately obvious. For that reason, problem or pathological gambling is often referred to as the "hidden addiction." Unlike substance abuse, for instance, where the impact of the behavior is generally immediately apparent—alcohol on the breath, red eyes, stumbling gait—gamblers can lose a great deal of money before anyone realizes there is a problem.

TEENS SPEAK

I Couldn't Seem to Stop

For me, the problem started so simply. A bunch of buddies and I were at one of our school's football games one night. A friend of mine said, "I betcha 10 bucks we lose the game." I said, "I'll take that bet, because you're crazy, there's no doubt that we're gonna win."

I was right. We won, and I felt great—not so much because the team had won, but because I had won the bet. From then on we bet at every game. I won more times than I lost.

Eventually, my buddy told me that I seemed to have a knack for picking a winner and suggested I try sports betting. He offered to hook me up with his bookie. The next week, I met up with the guy, placed some bets, and, again, I won more games than I lost.

It felt exhilarating to win, so the next week I upped the ante—I bet more money and bet on more games. This time, though, I lost more games than I won and ended up owing the bookie 50 bucks. After I paid up, I placed more bets hoping to recover the loss. But the next week I lost again. I continued to bet, but the more I tried to win, the more I seemed to lose.

Yet, I couldn't seem to stop. I kept thinking that if I kept betting, I would eventually score big, and then all my problems would be solved.

When I blew through my savings account and ran out of money, I began to steal from my family's business and family members. It took a while for them to realize that money was missing. When they asked me about the missing money, I lied and kept on stealing in order to continue betting. Eventually, they caught me red-handed, and I had to face the fact that I had a serious gambling problem.

When I started gambling, I didn't realize it would get the best of me. But it did. Not only did gambling get the best of me, but it also took the best from me. It turned me into a liar and a thief. What hurts most is that even though I haven't made a bet in over a year, I don't know if my family will ever truly trust me again.

Unfortunately, teen gambling can cause a great deal of damage well beyond the huge debt frequently incurred. All teen gambling—whether betting on sports using a **bookie,** playing poker for money with friends, or playing video gaming machines—is illegal. The consequences of underage gambling are ejection from the property, fines, or jail time. Adolescent gambling can also lead to academic problems including low or failing grades and truancy, job loss, physical difficulties associated with poor nutrition, and mental health disorders including, but not limited to, depression, anxiety, poor concentration, and exhaustion. Teen gamblers may lose their friends and develop strained relationships with their parents and siblings. Moreover, because gambling is often associated with criminal elements in society, teens who gamble may come in contact with organized crime and loan sharks only too willing to advance funds for gambling at astronomically high **interest rates.** To procure the funds needed to continue gambling, teens may also engage in stealing, drug dealing, or prostitution.

Q & A

Question: What are the signs of a gambling problem?

Answer: Below are some of the behaviors to look for:

- gambling until you lose all of your money
- losing sleep because you cannot stop thinking about gambling
- using your savings to continue gambling
- being unable to stop despite serious financial losses
- borrowing money or breaking the law, often stealing, to continue gambling
- feeling depressed or suicidal because of continued gambling
- gambling to win money to meet your financial requirements

Q & A

Question: What should I do if I think I have a gambling problem?

Answer: Talk to a trusted adult—a parent, a school counselor, a clergy member—and seek professional treatment. Problem or pathological gambling are treatable disorders.

See also: Addiction and Gambling; Alcohol, Drugs, and Gambling; Crime and Gambling; Risk Taking and Gambling; Youth at Special Risk

FURTHER READING
Johnson, Patrick B., and Micheline S. Malow-Iroff. *Adolescents and Risk: Making Sense of Adolescent Psychology.* Westport, Conn.: Praeger Publishers, 2008.
Shaffer, Howard J., Matthew N. Hall, and Joni Vander Bilt. *Futures at Stake: Youth, Gambling, and Society.* Reno: University of Nevada Press, 2003.

■ ADVERTISING AND GAMBLING

The influence on gambling behaviors of advertising, a form of communication intended to persuade an audience to purchase or take some action related to products, services, or ideas. Advertising raises people's awareness of products and services for the general purpose of increasing consumption. Also, its messages—communicated through TV, the Internet, film, music, and print—have the power of influencing social attitudes and values. Therefore, mass media is used to sell not only goods and services but also ideas: ideas about how one should behave, about what rules are important, about whom one should respect, and about what one should value. Advertising encourages individuals to make decisions and take actions that can result in both healthy and unhealthy outcomes.

A BRIEF HISTORY

In the 19th century, print was the primary medium for advertising. Then, as world economies expanded and technology advanced, advertising also grew. In the 1920s, the first radio stations were established, followed by the introduction of television in the late 1940s. Today, advertising appears most everywhere, including on mobile phone screens, buses, subway platforms, and cars. Advertising has developed into a billion-dollar industry on which many depend. In 2007, spending on advertising was estimated to exceed more than $150 billion in the United States and $385 billion worldwide.

GOOD AND BAD

Advertising is praised by some and criticized by others. While it can be seen as necessary for economic growth, advertising is not without its detractors and detriments. Some argue that advertising compromises individuality and independence by promoting conformity. It often appeals to emotion rather than rational thought. In fact, some critics argue that the most important element of advertising is not the provision of information but, rather, the manipulation of the mind through the use of psychological pressure. In other words, it has been argued that advertising exploits its audience by appealing to people's desires and fears. Many advertised products and services promise to fulfill the desires for happiness, health, fitness, appearance, self-esteem, belonging, social status, and wealth. Other messages promise to alleviate fears related to illness, aging, weakness, loneliness, and more.

Ironically, while commercialism increases, the visibility factor for any one single advertiser decreases. Therefore, in order to compete, the advertiser must make even greater efforts at exposure. For instance, until 1982, the prime-time television standard was no more than 9.5 minutes of advertising per hour. Today, TV commercials take up between 14 and 17 minutes of the hour, and advertising on the radio today accounts for approximately 19 minutes of the total broadcasting hour.

ADVERTISING AND SOCIAL PROBLEMS

While any attempt to restrict or ban advertising has been generally considered to be an attack on the fundamental right of free expression, according to the Constitution's First Amendment, advertising has been linked to a range of social problems. These include the growing problems of childhood obesity, underage drinking, underage gambling, and the development of problem and pathological gambling. As a result, there has been an increased effort to protect the public interest by regulating the content and influence of advertising, such as the ban of tobacco advertising on television.

The influence on gambling

Gambling advertising is controversial in many countries, including the United States. There is little doubt that advertising has played a role in the widespread cultural acceptance of gambling in this country.

Gambling advertising has created the perception that gambling, long considered a vice by many, is now a perfectly normal and socially acceptable form of entertainment for everyone. However, over the past several years, there has been considerable discussion about the influence of advertising on both the reported increases in underage gambling and the increased prevalence of problem and pathological gambling—in both adolescent and adult populations.

However, few researchers have examined the effect of gambling advertising on consumers. Also, the data from these studies have provided mixed results and inconclusive outcomes. For example, whereas two studies revealed that the behavior of a large number of problem gamblers was triggered by advertising, another study showed that its participants indicated advertising had little or nothing to with their gambling problem.

FACTORS THAT CAN TRIGGER PROBLEM GAMBLING

It has proven difficult to investigate the relationship between advertising and gambling, due to the complexities of the relationship itself. Although advertising may or may not play a role in the development of a gambling disorder, research has identified a number of individual and social factors related to problem or pathological gambling. These **triggers** exist mostly without the influence of advertising:

- sociological and demographic factors, such as low income, low education, being male
- friends who gamble and approve of gambling
- gambling at an early age
- a family history of problem gambling
- traumatic childhood experiences
- a strongly felt need for **dissociative** experiences
- **obsessive-compulsive disorder**
- age-related damage to certain parts of the brain
- preexisting alcohol or drug abuse or dependency.

Conversely, there are other factors commonly associated with the risk of developing a gambling problem that can be connected to gambling advertising. One such factor is availability. For example, gambling advertising

- informs and reminds consumers of the availability of gambling
- serves to recruit new players
- reminds established players to engage
- makes it more difficult for those with a gambling disorder to adhere to their decision to quit

While various groups, such as anti-gambling coalitions and religious organizations, argue that banning gambling advertising would be an appropriate step toward reducing gambling problems and its related consequences, others say that removing advertising will not stop people from gambling. They argue that anyone who wants to find an opportunity or place to gamble will do so—just as smokers continue to buy cigarettes despite the ban on television tobacco ads. Additionally, the history of gambling demonstrates that human beings in most cultures across space and time have been vulnerable to developing a problem with gambling well before the advent of advertising itself.

STATE-RUN LOTTERIES

While gambling advertising remains a controversial topic, even more controversial are state-run lotteries. Promoting gambling is different than merely permitting it. Operating a lottery places state governments in a new business, a business which they actively promote through advertising. According to the North American Association of State and Provincial Lotteries (NASPL), states spent $400 million in 1997 on lottery advertising, and that figure is likely higher today.

Additionally, according to a report published in 1999 by the U.S. National Gambling Impact Study Commission, one of the particularly troublesome components of lottery advertising was that much of it was misleading and deceptive. Some lottery advertisements contain statements that, if made by private businesses, could violate laws regarding truth in advertising. While the Federal Trade Commission requires statements about probability of winning in commercial sweepstakes games, there exists no such federal requirement for lotteries. In short, despite published advertising standards in 1999 that include being "truthful," lottery advertising rarely communicates the poor odds of winning; rather, the ads imply that the odds of winning are even "better than you think."

CODES OF CONDUCT

In 2003, the American Gaming Association (AGA), the casino industry's trade group, adopted a "Code of Conduct for Responsible Gaming." One section of the code pertains to advertising, stating that casinos must pledge to advertise responsibly by complying with all state and federal standards and refraining from making false or misleading claims. Also, to discourage underage gambling, casino advertising is not to do any of the following:

- contain cartoon figures, symbols, celebrity or entertainer endorsements, or language designed to appeal to underage gamblers, who, in most states, are those under 21
- feature current college athletes
- feature anyone who is or appears to be below the legal gambling age
- claim that gaming will guarantee an individual's social, financial, or personal success
- be placed in media specifically oriented to young people
- imply or suggest any illegal activity
- appear next to or near comics or other material that appeals to young people
- be placed at any venue where most of the audience is normally expected to be underage

Despite the presence of advertising codes, it is important to remember that, like most all other advertising, gambling advertising is biased. The tendency is to exaggerate winning and excitement, while minimizing the consequences—losing money, the possibility of developing a gambling problem, family issues, and more. Also, while at present it is not possible to determine whether gambling advertising leads to problem or pathological gambling, there is a general consensus between both gaming proponents and gambling critics that there must be a strong commitment to socially responsible gambling advertising.

See also: Addiction and Gambling; Adolescents and Gambling; Gambling, History of; Law and Gambling, The

FURTHER READING
Epstein, Lee, and Thomas G. Walker. *Constitutional Law for a Changing America: Institutional Powers and Constraints.* Washington, D.C.: CQ Press, 2010.
Ruschmann, Paul. *Legalized Gambling.* New York: Facts On File, 2009.

■ ALCOHOL, DRUGS, AND GAMBLING

The physical and psychological effects, especially on adolescents, of substance use and abuse, gambling, and other risk-taking activities. Adolescence and young adulthood are marked by changes in many areas of a young person's life. Along with the rapid biological and physical changes of **puberty**, there are important age-related tasks, transitions, and developments in social, emotional, and cognitive functioning. The ongoing developmental processes that begin in early adolescence include identity formation, increased autonomy and independence, a greater value of peer group relations, and enhanced perspective-taking and problem-solving skills.

INDEPENDENCE, STRESS, AND RISK TAKING

During adolescence, individuals generally begin to make independent decisions about their own behaviors, including making judgments about substance use (alcohol, drugs, tobacco), gambling, and other risk-taking activities. These decisions occur at a time when adolescents are highly susceptible to external influences such as societal messages, media portrayals, adult role models, and peer pressure. Each or all of these influences may promote substance use, gambling, and other risk-taking behaviors as a way for an adolescent to appear mature, rebellious, and independent.

While most behaviors typically begin and develop within the context of family, society, and culture, there are also personal and internal factors that increase an adolescent's vulnerability for risk taking. These factors include low self-esteem, mood instability, and underdeveloped levels of self-discipline. Furthermore, many experts believe that the severity of risk-taking behaviors in adolescence is associated with increased stress, a naturally occurring accompaniment to multiple adolescent developmental processes, and either a deficiency in the number of coping skills necessary to deal with negative life events or an overall general inability to cope with negative life events. From this perspective then, risk-taking behaviors, including substance use and gambling, may become a poorly thought out solution or a coping response to difficult life situations.

Patterns of risk-taking behaviors

No one pattern of substance use or risk-taking behavior can fully account for all individuals. However, the general pattern includes

- initiation or experimental use or behavior during early adolescence
- a rapid increase in use or behavior during adolescence
- a peak during young adulthood
- a more or less gradual decline through the remainder of adulthood

An individual's pattern of substance use and risk-taking behavior is typically shaped by a series of transitions, goals, and milestones that occur during an adolescent's years of rapid developmental change.

Commonly used substances

Alcohol, tobacco, and marijuana are the most commonly used substances among both adolescents and adults in the United States. While alcohol and tobacco are both legal substances, marijuana generally is not, except in some states where it is available for certain medical uses. Non-medical pill use, defined as the abuse of prescription psychotherapeutics or prescription **stimulants**, is the second most prevalent type of illicit drug use after marijuana. Other illicit substances used by adolescents include heroin, cocaine, and amphetamines; however, while teen alcohol use continues to rise, there has been a gradual decline over the past several years in the use of these illegal substances among secondary school students.

While the majority of individuals who experiment with risk-taking behaviors—specifically alcohol, other drugs, and gambling—experience no significant consequences, some individuals develop serious problems including those related to substance and behavioral abuse and dependency issues. A problem exists when someone continues to drink alcohol, take drugs, and/or gamble even when these behaviors cause trouble in the person's life. These troubles may occur in school and/or work performance, in social and/or family relationships,

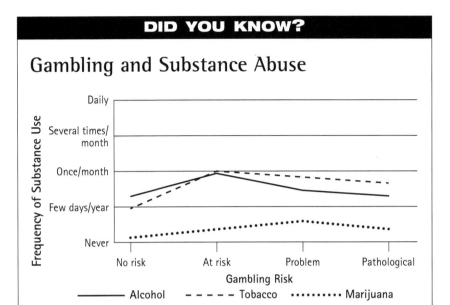

DID YOU KNOW?

Gambling and Substance Abuse

Gambling on all levels (at risk, problem, and pathological) is on the rise in the United States and often occurs along with other addictive risky behaviors. A 2006 study of 3,596 participants living in New Mexico found that the average frequency of alcohol consumption is highest among those at risk for problem gambling and lowest among pathological gamblers. The average frequency of tobacco use is highest among at-risk gamblers with a decline in the problem among pathological gamblers. Marijuana use is highest among problem and pathological gamblers.

Source: Sandra L. Momper, Jorge Delva, Andrew Grogran-Kaylor, Ninive Sanchez, and Rachel A. Volberg. "The Association of At-Risk, Problem, and Pathological Gambling with Substance Use, Depression, and Arrest History," *Journal of Gambling* 24 (July 2010).

physical and/or mental health, problems with the law, finances, and general self-concept. These problems associated with alcohol, other drugs, and/or gambling usually develop gradually, over time. The more an individual drinks, takes drugs, or gambles, the greater his or her risk for abusing the substance or behavior and becoming dependent on or addicted to it.

MORE THAN ONE DISORDER

A significant problem that involves two or more co-occurring disorders—such as alcohol, drugs, and gambling—is called **comorbidity**.

There are three ways to imagine the causal relationship between pathological gambling and other disorders:

1. problem gambling as a direct cause of a secondary order, for example, substance abuse/dependence
2. problem gambling as a direct result of another more primary disorder, for example, substance abuse/dependence
3. problem gambling as just one of a number of disorders with a common cause or common causes

Although the developmental order of comorbid problems is not well understood, some researchers have suggested that disordered gambling may serve as a **gateway** to substance abuse or dependence. Experts have shown that excessive gambling among adolescents has been associated with increased alcohol and other substance use disorders, higher rates of depression and **anxiety,** increased thoughts of suicide and suicide attempts, and increased delinquency and criminal behavior. Furthermore, young people who are in psychiatric hospitals, chemical dependency programs, and juvenile detention centers display gambling rates that are approximately double that of adolescents from school or community samples.

Gateway drugs and behaviors

There is also a large body of research that suggests that it is substance use that may serve as the gateway for the development of a gambling disorder, not the other way around. Research results indicate that for most gamblers with comorbid disorders, the onset of substance abuse or dependency preceded their gambling problem. In these cases, alcohol was the most commonly used substance, followed by marijuana and cocaine. Additionally, nicotine dependence also often co-occurs with pathological gambling. The results of one study found that 60 percent of those diagnosed with pathological gambling were also diagnosed with a dependence on nicotine.

Fact Or Fiction

A cigarette is not a gateway drug.

The Facts: Nicotine products such as cigarettes or chewing tobacco are indeed gateway drugs and can lead to using other drugs or to illegal activities. In fact, recent studies have shown that nicotine leads to a higher percentage of drug use or risky behavior than does marijuana.

Regardless of the order of onset, data reveal that when an individual develops either a substance use disorder or a gambling disorder, he or she becomes vulnerable to developing the other. Both disorders share developmental commonalities and devastating outcomes. While gambling behaviors have been shown to begin earlier than most other potentially addictive behaviors, including the abuse of tobacco, alcohol and/or other drugs, both gambling and substance use usually begin in adolescence or early adulthood and follow similar stages of progressions. Essentially, both disorders share these determinants:

- physiological predisposition
- psychological processes
- environmental stressors
- social and familial influences

Similar criteria

Pathological gambling was initially introduced in the *Diagnostic and Statistical Manual of Mental Disorders (DSM)* as a disorder of impulse control, not elsewhere classified. Although it remains in the impulse control disorders section, many of the diagnostic criteria overlap with those of substance use disorders. Specifically, there are 10 compulsive gambling criteria listed, five of which parallel substance use disorder criteria:

1. preoccupation with gambling/substance
2. a need to increase the size or frequency of bets/substance use (tolerance)
3. repeated efforts to stop or cut down gambling/substance use
4. restlessness and irritability if not gambling/using the substance or prevented from gambling/using the substance (withdrawal)
5. forgoing social, work/academic, or recreational activities in order to gamble/use the substance

Although pathological gambling and substance use disorders are classified differently in the *DSM,* many scientists have long believed that gambling disorders closely resemble substance use disorders not only on the outside, but, increasingly, on the inside as well. A growing body of research demonstrates, to varying degrees, that gambling has the capacity to mimic the subjective effects of ingesting psychoactive drugs. Brain imaging and neurochemical tests have provided some convincing evidence that gambling behaviors activate the brain's reward system in much the same way as a drug does. For example, neuroscientists have shown that the central nervous system reward circuits for winning money parallel the reward mechanisms associated with the anticipation of cocaine use. Furthermore, some investigators have speculated that pathological gambling and substance use disorders may have similar underlying **neurotransmitter** deficits. The link with **dopamine** may be of greatest interest due to its association with reward and reinforcement processes. **Serotonin** is also of interest because low levels of this neurotransmitter have been linked to **impulsive** behaviors.

Similar treatment

Pathological gambling and substance use disorders also share treatment approaches. Many of the treatment interventions applied to pathological gambling were adapted from substance use disorder treatment theories and models. Also, Gamblers Anonymous, the self-help group, was modeled after **Alcoholics Anonymous (AA).**

HOW CAN YOU TELL?

Identifying a problem is the first step in dealing with it. The following checklists can be of help.

Checklist for Alcohol or Other Drug Use

___Your use of alcohol/drugs has increased.

___You drink/use to get through new situations or social occasions.

___You cannot remember things you said or did while drinking/using.

___You cover up or lie about your alcohol/drug use.

___You have problems at school/work or miss school/work because of your alcohol/drug use.

___You have arguments with friends and/or family members because of your alcohol/drug use.

___Your alcohol/drug use is causing financial problems.

___You have legal problems because of your alcohol/drug use.

___You have tried to cut down or stop but could not.

___You have broken promises to others because of your drinking/drug use.

___Someone has told you that they are concerned about your drinking/drug use.

Checklist for Problem Gambling

___You are placing larger bets and/or betting more often.

___You have growing debt problems because of your gambling.

___You hope for the "big win" to solve your financial or other problems.

___You spend large amounts of time gambling, leaving little time for family, friends, or other interests.

___You have tried to cut back or stop gambling but have not been able to do so.

___You lie or cover up your gambling.

___You have feelings of "highs and lows" and miss the thrill of gambling when you cannot gamble.

If you answered *yes* to any of the statements in the above checklists, you may have an alcohol, drug, and/or gambling problem. If you think you have a problem with alcohol, other drugs, and/or gambling, talk to a trusted adult—a parent, a school counselor, a clergy member—and seek professional assistance. Treatment is available.

See also: Addiction and Gambling; Adolescents and Pathological Gambling; Depression and Gambling; Family Life and Gambling; Peer Pressure and Gambling; Risk Taking and Gambling; Youth at Special Risk

FURTHER READING
Petry, N. "Gambling and Substance Use Disorders: Current Status and Future Directions." *The American Journal on Addiction* 16 (2007).

Scheier, L. *Handbook of Drug Use Etiology: Theory, Methods, and Empirical Findings*. Washington, D.C.: American Psychological Association, 2010.

■ BINGE GAMBLING

Excessive gambling that is driven by impulsivity and **compulsion.** Binges are periods or bouts, usually brief, of overindulgence and are seen also in eating, drinking alcoholic beverages, and other compulsive behaviors.

Individuals who have difficulty controlling their gambling urges experience different levels of problematic gambling behavior. For example, binge gamblers may fit the medical criteria for pathological gambling only while bingeing but not when they are in a dormant stage. Binge gamblers present irregular, uncontrolled episodes of gambling, while the majority of the time they remain abstinent from any form of gambling. This subgroup of pathological or problem gamblers has not yet been identified in the *Diagnostic and Statistical Manual of Mental Disorders IV—Text Revision (DSM-IV-TR)*.

DEFINING THE BINGE CONCEPT

Binge drinking and binge eating are disorders that have been heavily researched, unlike binge gambling. However, binge gambling is similar to binge eating or drinking. According to M. Griffiths in an article for *The Psychologist*, "Internet Addiction: Fact or Fiction?," "loss of control, salience, mood modification, conflict, withdrawal symptoms, denial, etc.," are symptoms related to binge behaviors. Also, in 2006, researchers L. Nower and A. Blaszczynski published a report in *International Gambling Studies* outlining six factors that differentiate binge gamblers and pathological gamblers. These include

1. impulsive onset of irregular periods of persistent gambling
2. spending large amounts of income
3. spending large amounts of money in a small time frame
4. feeling compelled and out of control in relation to gambling
5. exhibiting a striking sense of distress

6. showing a lack of worry and urges to gamble in between bouts of gambling

In a case study, Griffiths describes that a motivation to gamble appears to be related to low self-esteem, depression, and a great deal of unstructured time. Problem gamblers, including binge gamblers, use gambling as a way to feel better when their mood is less than ideal. However, after a gambling session, they tend to feel worse than before because of their monetary loss.

Binge drinking
Binge drinking is the consumption of large amounts of alcohol, about five drinks for males and four drinks for females, per one drinking episode. The difference between males and females is due to different body mass and metabolic rates. A person is considered a binge drinker if he or she has had "three or more binges in the past two weeks." Although binge drinking has not yet been recognized in the *DSM-IV-TR*, which means these individuals might or might not fit the criteria for alcohol dependence, there are thought to be long-term effects. Animal studies suggest that young binge drinkers—college students and adolescents—may be at risk of developing memory impairment in their adulthood.

Binge eating
Binge eating is defined by the *DSM-IV-TR* as "eating in a discrete period of time an amount of food that is definitely larger than most people would eat in a similar period of time under similar circumstances," and it occurs with a loss of control over eating during that bout. Binge eating disorder is characterized as having no control over the amount and cessation of the consumption of food while experiencing the binge, including the following factors as described in the *DSM-IV-TR*:

1. eating faster than normal
2. eating until painfully full
3. eating larger than normal amounts of food while not being physically hungry
4. having a preference of eating alone due to pure embarrassment over the amount of food consumed; and finally

5. feeling revolted, depressed, and embarrassed after the binge-eating episode

In a recent study, researchers found that binge eaters are twice as likely to experience another disorder at the same time, such as co-occurrence with alcohol and/or anxiety/depressive disorders. Also, they are four times as likely to experience **panic attacks**. Additionally, physical deterioration is a common factor among binge eaters: they usually report limb or joint pain, headaches, gastrointestinal and menstrual problems, breathing problems, and even chest pain.

Similarities between other binge disorders and binge gambling

Binge gambling is similar to the concepts of binge drinking and binge eating. These gamblers experience frequent bouts of excessive gambling without being able to control their behavior. However, they also have periods of time without any preoccupation related to gambling, meaning that their gambling may not produce a problem at all. Binge gamblers do not necessarily fit the criteria for pathological gamblers because their symptoms are not persistent but only sporadic and temporary, dependent on triggers. As a result, binge gamblers usually go undiagnosed and untreated.

Like pathological gamblers, binge gamblers' episodes can be triggered by distress, such as unresolved issues in relationships, work, school, and their social environment. They cope with these stressors by binge gambling. Binge gamblers also are likely to experience financial hardships. However, unlike pathological gamblers, they do not experience a constant preoccupation with gambling.

BIOLOGICAL FACTORS

Although it is true that external factors appear to be the main triggers of a binge gambling episode, there are also biological factors related to specific brain activity that is linked to pathological gambling and that one can speculate is also related to binge gambling. According to researchers Moreno, Saiz-Ruiz, and López-Ibor, **serotonergic dysfunction** has been found to be related to poor impulse control disorders, such as pathological gambling. In addition, other researchers have found that **noradrenergic** and **dopaminergic dysfunction**s are biological causes of pathological gambling. This appears to be related to a lower serotonin activity and to a lower than normal serotonin availability. Serotonin is the neurotransmitter that affects a person's moods or feelings. There also is evidence that, in binge disorders, there is a decrease in the platelet monomine oxidase B (MAO-B), which is responsible for metabolizing hormones among other activities in the body.

Q & A

Question: Does binge gambling lead to pathological gambling?

Answer: Yes, even though binge gambling occurs in spurts, these spurts can last hours or days. The physiological and psychological effects of the binges can lead to a serious and lasting gambling problem.

PERSONALITY TRAITS

Impulsivity is a main factor in many impulse control disorders, such as binge drinking, binge eating, and problem and pathological gambling, which may include binge gambling. Signs of impulsivity include

- a sense of urgency related to behaviors
- lack of planning
- lack of perseverance
- a strong sense of sensation-seeking behavior or the pursuit of novel stimuli

However, the research does not yet explain how binge gamblers experience impulsivity during the periods in which their gambling is under control. More research is certainly needed.

Although binge gambling currently lacks the research and diagnostic criteria of other binge behaviors, binge gamblers usually fit the criteria of pathological gamblers while experiencing a binge, which is usually triggered by distress and even by biological functions. Also, in addition to gambling and losing significant amounts of money that will burden their quality of life, binge gamblers' relationships with others, especially those close to them, are likely to suffer. These gamblers will experience guilt, depression, and embarrassment due to their gambling episodes.

Individuals with a binge gambling problem can benefit from seeking help to cease or control their gambling, and a great start would be Gamblers Anonymous. This self-help group offers social support from other individuals experiencing similar struggles.

See also: Addiction and Gambling; Adolescents and Gambling; Alcohol, Drugs, and Gambling; Gender and Gambling; Help for Gamblers

FURTHER READING

American Psychiatric Association. *Diagnostic and Statistical Manual of Mental Disorders IV–Text Revision.* Washington, D.C.: American Psychiatric Association, 2000.

Moreno, I., J. Saiz-Ruiz, and J. J. López-Ibov. "Serotonin and Gambling Dependence." *Human Psychopharmacology: Clinical and Experimental* 6, Supp. 1 (October 1991): S9–S12.

■ CRIME AND GAMBLING

Illegal acts—such as theft, assault, homicide, or illicit drug use—which are thought to be associated with gambling. For a long time gambling was illegal. Any person participating in the activity was guilty of committing a crime and could face time in prison. Today, gambling is legal in most countries throughout the world and in every state in the United States except Utah and Hawaii.

Laws about gambling are not consistent throughout the world nor are they the same in every state. Although some forms of gambling are illegal, and therefore engaging in them is committing a crime, most crimes associated with gambling are not gambling itself.

TYPES OF CRIMINAL ACTIVITY

Some of the crimes associated with gambling are assault, theft and robbery, money laundering, and even murder. Many cities and states do not want **casinos** built on their land due to the anticipated increase in criminal activities. This controversial subject has sparked much debate among policy makers and led to recent research on gambling and crime.

Recent studies

The United States Department of Justice has examined numerous studies on the relationship of crime and gambling, looking especially at those who have been arrested and imprisoned and how their arrests relate to problem and pathological gambling. One study found pathological gambling to be 3–5 percent more prevalent in arrestees than the general population. The same study found that one-third of the prison population who had been identified as pathological gamblers had committed robbery for gambling purposes within the past year, and 13 percent had committed assault.

In another study, which focused on the prison population in Las Vegas, Nevada, and Des Moines, Iowa, researchers found the following:

- 14.2 percent of arrestees in Las Vegas and 9.2 percent in Des Moines were pathological gamblers. This is important because, in contrast, the prevalence of pathological gamblers in the general population is 1–3 percent.

- 30 percent of all pathological gamblers arrested in Des Moines and Las Vegas had committed robbery. Most of the arrestees stated that the robbery arrest was related to stealing money for gambling.

- 13 percent of the same population assaulted another individual during the robbery.

Addiction and crime

Gambling has been linked to addiction and the property and violent crimes committed under the influence of drugs, alcohol, or a combination of the two. Many casinos offer free drinks to patrons who play machines or table games. If an individual is a pathological gambler who drinks while playing, there is a good chance that he or she has a comorbid addiction.

Drug abuse and addiction have also been associated with gambling. For example, individuals may use drugs to escape the depression linked to the lying, stealing, and material loss that accompany pathological gambling. Losing friends, money, and family leads to depression, and, to feel better, many people self-medicate with illicit drugs or the abuse of prescription drugs. In a recent study of prison inmates, for example, more than 60 percent of all pathological gamblers tested positive for abused drugs.

Gambling is also linked to the illegal sale of drugs. Although studies have not shown a distinct correlation between drug dealing and gambling, many cities refuse to build casinos within their limits because of the fear of drug sales, robbery, and assault. Officials and citizens are afraid that gamblers will resort to selling drugs for money.

The theory has some basis. In a recent study, interviewers found that more than 20 percent of all gamblers in the prison system have sold drugs to acquire money for gambling.

Fact Or Fiction?

All pathological gamblers commit crimes.

The Facts: While not all pathological gamblers commit crimes, many do resort to robbery and drug-dealing to pay their gambling debts and/or come up with more money to continue gambling.

ADOLESCENT GAMBLING AND CRIME

In most states, gambling is illegal for anyone under the age of 21. (In 11 states and in Washington, D.C., the legal gambling age is 18.) Online gambling sites, which are governed by different laws, also allow individuals as young as 18 to play. However, a lot of sites will not permit anyone under 21 to collect his or her winnings. Because adolescents tend to be drawn to high-risk situations, which are potentially exciting, they are at a high risk for developing a gambling problem. Gambling may seem thrilling and "cool" at first, but it can lead to more severe risk-taking scenarios.

Adolescent theft

Many teenagers fall prey to the negative activities associated with gambling. Because most adolescents do not have full-time jobs, those who gamble will look for other ways to find money. This can lead to stealing from family, friends, and employers. Peer pressure also may lead to theft in order to gamble. Stealing money is a serious offense and can be prosecuted, even if a person steals from someone he or she knows. Not only can the crime lead to time in a juvenile detention center, or prison, depending on the laws of the state in which the offense occurs, but it also can break people's trust. Theft also can result in larger-scale, violent crimes, such as assault and robbery.

Adolescent addiction

Gambling is also linked to drug and alcohol abuse. Using illegal drugs is a crime in the United States for everyone, regardless of age. Often, stimulants such as cocaine (which is highly addictive) or methamphetamine and amphetamines (which are known to increase aggression) are used by gamblers to stay awake during episodes of play. Adolescents may also turn to drug dealing to try to recoup money lost while gambling.

Alcohol, which is often available to gamblers, is illegal to any individual under the age of 21. Underage drinkers can be cited with a ticket or sent to a juvenile detention center. Also, adults who supply alcohol to underage individuals face even harsher charges.

MONEY PROBLEMS AND GAMBLING

Gambling often results in the loss of a great deal of money. To ensure their success, casinos and online gambling sites employ a **house advantage**. The house advantage is a percentage equation that works against the gambler. For every dollar the gambler plays, the house, or casino, takes a certain percentage. The percentage may change from game to game, anywhere from .5 percent to 20 percent. Simply put, casino and online games are created to make a profit. This makes it difficult for anyone to make money by gambling.

"Chasing the loss"

Because gambling incurs frequent losses, individuals feel compelled to "chase their loss." Gamblers convince themselves that they need to play for more and more money to make up for their losses. Most of the time, pathological gamblers are not expecting to win large amounts of money to use for recreation; instead, they are playing only to pay off their gambling debt.

Loss of trust

Gamblers usually borrow money from friends and family, a habit that can result in a loss of trust and the inability to repay those people. Borrowing money from family can be not only embarrassing but often also leads to lying. The gambler falsely imagines that he or she will spend the money gambling, win, and then be able to pay back the debt. This rarely happens; instead the gambler moves from friend to friend, family member to family member, trying the system over and over again. Eventually, the lies do not work, and the gambler suffers the loss of trust from family and the loss of friends.

DEBT AND CREDIT

Many casinos and online gambling sites allow users to buy markers with credit cards, thereby often incurring extremely high levels of

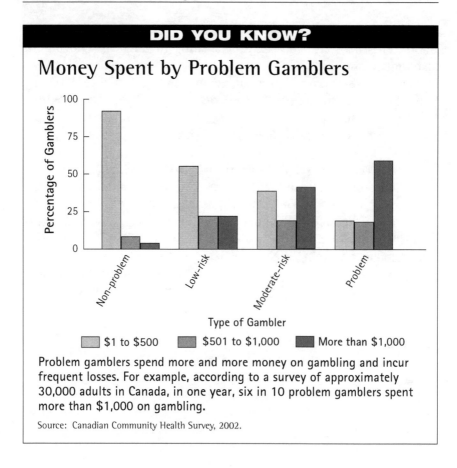

DID YOU KNOW?

Money Spent by Problem Gamblers

Problem gamblers spend more and more money on gambling and incur frequent losses. For example, according to a survey of approximately 30,000 adults in Canada, in one year, six in 10 problem gamblers spent more than $1,000 on gambling.

Source: Canadian Community Health Survey, 2002.

debt. Credit cards usually have high spending limits and even higher interest rates. Because interest charges accrue at lightning speed, the gambler ends up spending more than originally intended. Also, if a card is not paid off on time, the interest rate goes up, and if even more time elapses since payment has been made, the individual's account may be sent to a collection service. Being sent to collection tarnishes a person's credit score for several years and impacts one's ability to purchase a car or house, or even take out a student loan.

Casinos often give gamblers a line of credit with which to play. The line of credit is to be paid back before any winnings can be collected. However, the player often is unable to win enough to pay back the amount of the credit, or loan. When this happens, casinos can press charges to collect their losses. This is often a felony offense, and the penalty may include time in jail.

More problems

On occasion, someone close to a gambler pays off the person's gambling debt, which is known as a bailout. Most gambling treatment programs do not support bailouts, because gamblers who are bailed out return to gambling at higher rates than those who work to pay off their debts. Pathological gamblers often accrue an amount of debt in the thousands. Gambling debt is typically the cause of depression and other mental health disorders, physical health problems, family disputes and estrangement, and job loss.

See also: Addiction and Gambling; Adolescents and Gambling; Law and Gambling, The

FURTHER READING

Ashcroft, J., D. J. Daniels, and S. V. Hart. *Gambling and Crime Among Arrestees: Exploring the Link.* U.S. Department of Justice, 2004.

Humphrey, Hale. *This Must Be Hell: A Look at Pathological Gambling.* Bloomington, Ind.: iUniverse, 2009.

■ DEPRESSION AND PATHOLOGICAL GAMBLING

The relationship between excessive problem gambling and the mental condition that causes feelings of profound sadness and hopelessness. It is difficult to determine whether depression is a symptom of gambling or a consequence. It is possible that a gambler begins to experience depression after realizing the amount of money he or she has lost. Often, pathological gamblers lose all of their belongings and acquire debts that they cannot pay back. Upon realizing this situation, the gambler can become depressed and develop a sense of helplessness. This in turn can lead to a deeper level of depression.

Alternately, a gambler utilizes gaming as a means to treat his or her existing depression. In this case, the gaming is a symptom of the depression. The depressed person might gamble in order to add some excitement to life. He or she might find a thrill in the occasional wins or even the "chase" of lost money. Ultimately, the thrill is only a temporary relief or distraction from the symptoms of depression.

GAMBLING AND ADDICTION

Some studies suggest that people who suffer from depression and use gaming as a kind of treatment can become addicted to gaming, unable to stop despite negative outcomes. These people are ultimately conditioning themselves to depend on the rush of winning. Over time, the amount of money gambled, and lost, increases, resulting possibly from the fact that they can no longer obtain a thrill from gambling small amounts of money.

Overall, whether the depression is a symptom or a consequence of the excessive gaming, it is important to seek treatment for both disorders. This begins by understanding the disorders and the impact they have on a person.

SYMPTOMS OF DEPRESSION

Clinical or serious depression is a disorder characterized by loss of interest or pleasure, persistent poor mood, loss of weight, insomnia or hypersomnia, psychomotor agitation or retardation, fatigue, feelings of worthlessness, excessive or inappropriate guilt, trouble concentrating, suicidal thoughts, and preoccupation with death.

Q & A

Question: Is depression normal?

Answer: Everyone can experience a mild form of depression, which can be triggered in many ways—by the death of a loved one, loss of a job, termination of a relationship, and any stressful situation. Typically, however, normal episodes of depression last a few days and are not severe enough to interfere, except briefly, with daily activities.

Major or prolonged depression is not normal, and it affects all aspects of a person's life. In contrast to the depression we all can experience, individuals with clinical or major depression have episodes that can last weeks, months, or even years. Typically, people with depressive disorder have more bad days than good days. On average, if a person is not treated, the depressive episode can last four months or longer. Depression is one of the most debilitating disorders and can be very costly. In fact, suicide can result from long periods of depression, especially if untreated.

People who suffer from depression can see their lives being affected in many ways. Typically, they lose interest or pleasure in all activities, even the one they used to enjoy the most. Long periods of depression can severely affect daily functioning and can lead to failure or persistent poor grades in school, job loss, termination of relationships, distancing from others, and guilt.

Dual diagnosis

Depressed individuals who are also pathological gamblers tend to distance themselves from family and friends. One explanation for this behavior is that these individuals lose interest in others because they are too preoccupied with gambling. Without friends or family, the individual is also without a support system. This in turn can negatively affect any treatment process. Furthermore, losing one's support system can lead to a deeper level of depression.

Risk of suicide

Suicide can result from prolonged depression. Individuals with depression frequently have thoughts of death or attempt suicide. These people typically believe that they will be doing others a favor by dying, that this will prevent further problems for their loved ones. Moreover, they often believe that suicide is the answer to their emotional and physical sufferings.

Prolonged depression is not uncommon among problem gamblers. Research has shown that female gamblers are typically more prone to depression and suicidal ideation than are males. However, males have the highest completion rate in suicide attempts. Often, a suicide is completed because of impulsive tendencies and aggressive behaviors, which are higher in boys and men. A report published in 2010 in the *Journal of Affective Disorders* and other studies indicate that, on average, 15 percent of individuals with major depression disorder are successful at suicide. Other studies indicate that up to 90 percent of people who die by suicide were suffering from a mental-health issue, such as depression or substance abuse.

Suicide is frequently triggered by the guilt, shame, and preoccupations that arise from gambling. An individual who cannot find a solution for the financial burden he or she has created may think that suicide is the best option. Moreover, pathological gamblers often become physically and psychologically exhausted from the lying, cheating, and committing of illegal acts and from the emotional, physical, and economic

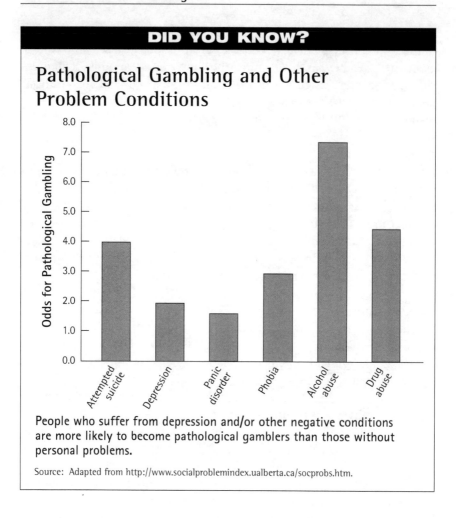

DID YOU KNOW?

Pathological Gambling and Other Problem Conditions

People who suffer from depression and/or other negative conditions are more likely to become pathological gamblers than those without personal problems.

Source: Adapted from http://www.socialproblemindex.ualberta.ca/socprobs.htm.

losses. The exhaustion can lead individuals to contemplate suicide as the escape from their problems. Suicide, however, is the most preventable death, because most people do not want to die.

TREATMENT OF CO-OCCURRING DISORDERS

Research shows that an effective way to treat individuals with both depression and pathological gambling is to incorporate **cognitive behavioral therapy (CBT)** into their treatment. The goal of CBT is to help an individual change his or her behavior by learning new coping skills for symptoms of depression and gambling impulses. In other words, a therapist retrains a person's brain by teaching him or her new ways of coping with the anxiety, impulses, negative thoughts, guilt, anger, and other implications of these disorders.

Typically, with CBT, a person benefits from learning techniques that can help him or her release uncomfortable or painful feelings. For example, therapy might target the irrational beliefs associated with gambling, such as the idea of "chasing" losses, which is the misguided belief that the gambler has a system that eventually will pay off. Identifying triggers for their behaviors and learning coping skills for those triggers is another way to treat impulsivity.

Challenging beliefs and behaviors is also important in treating pathological gambling. This can be done by helping a person see his or her reality. Other tools of the therapist and support groups are sincerity, unconditional positive regard, and empathy.

See also: Addiction and Gambling; Alcohol, Drugs, and Gambling; Family Life and Gambling; Prevention and Intervention; Protective Factors; Public Health Issues and Gambling; Suicide and Gambling

FURTHER READING

Ladouceur, Robert, Caroline Sylvain, Claude Boutin, and Celine Doucet. *Understanding and Treating the Pathological Gambler.* New York: John Wiley & Sons, 2002.

Wong, Paul W. C., Wincy S. C. Chan, Yeates Conwell, Kenneth R. Cooner, and Paul S. F. Yip. "A Psychological Autopsy Study of Pathological Gamblers Who Died by Suicide." *Journal of Affective Disorders* 120 (2010): 213–216.

■ FAMILY LIFE AND GAMBLING

The effects of problem gambling on the entire family, especially those living in the household. When a parent has a problem with gambling, he or she is not the only one who is negatively impacted: children may experience a very difficult and unstable family environment.

The nuclear family—traditionally two parents and their unmarried children—can be affected on many different levels, such as harsh financial strains, legal problems, and deterioration of physical and psychological health that are due to losses in different areas of the family's life. The spouse and children of a problem gambler are usually unaware of the extent of the problem until it is severe.

The *Diagnostic and Statistical Manual of Mental Disorders, DSM-IV-TR,* describes pathological gambling as a behavior that has become a severe problem for an individual. Researchers believe that about 1 million people, about 1 percent of the population, fall in this category in the United States, and about 4 to 6 million people, 2 to 3 percent of the U.S. population, have a less than severe problem with gambling. What does that mean for us? Simply, it means that individuals who are gambling are no longer doing it for fun and that it is now an uncontrollable problem. With such large numbers of people experiencing gambling problems, it follows that families are experiencing the negative consequences of the gamblers' behavior. However, because the person with a gambling problem usually hides his or her actions due to shame and guilt, the family members are often unaware of the cause of their problems. In addition, problem gambling is usually accompanied by other issues, such as depression, suicide attempts, substance abuse, antisocial personality disorder, and a history of negative family experiences.

IMPACT ON THE GAMBLER

The individual who is unable to control his or her gambling is very likely to experience many other life problems, such as stress-related physical problems, emotional issues within his or her relationship, and financial strain. As reported in the *Journal of Gambling Studies,* Valerie C. Lorenz and Robert A. Yaffee studied the impact of gambling among those attending self-help groups. They discovered that gamblers are prone to suffer from stomach ailments, sleeping problems, and depression. Also, problem gamblers usually come from families in which they suffered some trauma and in which it was very likely that one of the parents also had problem gambling issues.

Generally, the quality of life in the family of a gambler is far from healthy because of all the negative consequences that the gambler experiences from his or her behavior. Also, problem gambling may be a reflection of modeled behavior from the gambler's family of origin.

IMPACT ON THE SPOUSE OR PARTNER

Relationships can be challenging, but they are even more challenging if one of the partners is experiencing a problem with gambling. Spouses of individuals with problems gambling are usually unaware of the problem because the gambler hides the intensity of the problem as long as possible, until he or she can no longer hide it and must admit it. The spouse usually describes this confession as "traumatic," because the spouse had no idea that the problem existed and cannot believe that his or her partner was able to hide it for such a long time. The spouse usually experiences stress in social, psychological, and economic areas of his or her life. After discovering the problem gambling, the spouse typically takes on responsibility for household finances, which means that he or she also will be likely to take on the stressful responsibility of communicating with all the creditors to whom her partner owes money.

Spouses of problem gamblers also usually experience poor physical health related to stress, chronic and constant headaches, breathing difficulties, backaches, stomach problems, high blood pressure, insomnia, and asthma. In addition, spouses also experience intense emotional consequences, such as depression, anxiety, anger, isolation, and suicide. Spouses or partners are more likely to experience intimate partner violence and other problems in the relationship, and couples in which one partner is a problem gambler are more likely to separate and eventually divorce.

THE IMPACT OF GAMBLING ON THE CHILDREN

The children living in a household affected by problem gambling suffer a lot, because they are frequent witnesses of unhealthy family interactions, are the victims of abuse, receive less than ideal emotional support from immediate and extended family members, and have negative role models. According to Lorenz, children might be the most victimized by the illness. Here are reasons why children with a parent affected by problem gambling are more likely to behave in negative ways:

- They have yet to learn how to solve problems with others.
- They do not know how to reduce stress or tension.
- They have not learned how to cope with issues that might come up in school with friends or in the family.

These children are also more likely to behave in negative ways during their adult years and themselves become gamblers. Researchers state that children with a parent with problem gambling will suffer from what they call "pervasive loss," the loss of the gambling parent in a physical and emotional way; the loss of the relationship that is supposed to provide security, trust, and stability; the loss of connecting with extended family members; and the loss of benefits that money can bring, including sometimes the family house.

Emotional losses due to gambling

Pervasive losses are experienced at different levels, related to the ever present gambling activities and the constant tension between the gambler and non-gambler parents. The emotional loss experienced by the children results from

- the problem gambler parent's not being the same type of person he or she used to be
- the parent's not being there to support and express his or her love
- the loss of trust from all the broken promises, such as failing to come and visit at a certain day and time, after parents have separated, and not following through
- the loss of stability, security, and connection with the rest of the extended family

Children in the Dayshire studies described their gambling parent as "deceptive, unreliable, irresponsible, irrational, uninterested, and selfish." Children also miss school-related and recreational activities because of the lack of money; the losses are not only physical and emotional, but also material, such as the loss of the family home, savings, and appropriate amounts of food to eat.

Other negative outcomes

Children of a problem gambler usually begin to assume an adult role in order to compensate for the lack of contribution to the family by the gambling parent; at the same time, they also tend to suffer from emotional and physical abuse, which can be violent. They also often suffer from role confusion as they become involuntarily entangled in the problems of their parents. Some children even express that they feel guilty and responsible for their current family environment. Several studies have found that children suffer the most from the negative family environment because they feel "abandoned, rejected, neglected, emotionally deprived, angry, hurt, sad, confused, isolated and/or guilty, helpless, anxious, and depressed." In fact, some researchers have revealed that these children are sometimes locked in vehicles by the problem gambler outside gambling establishments. In addition to the psychological damage that the children of problem gamblers experience, they are also prone to suffer from stress-induced illnesses and begin to smoke, drink, use drugs, suffer from compulsive eating, and even begin gambling because of the accumulation of risk factors over their developing years.

HOPE FOR FAMILIES WITH A PATHOLOGICAL GAMBLER

Although children, the spouse, and even the gambler suffer from the negative family environment, there is hope. Self-help groups, such as Gamblers Anonymous, provide social support for the gambler and for the family members, at Gam-Anon. Although these groups are great in finding people to whom the families can relate, professional therapy is essential for recovery, especially therapy with a focus on the family as a whole. In family therapy, members might be able not only to uncover underlying issues that might trigger gambling but they also might be able to relate to each other in a healthier way.

Fact Or Fiction?

If someone in my family gambles, it's his problem.

The Facts: Some therapists specialize in family counseling because problem gambling affects a lot more people than just the gambler. You also can get help by attending Gamblers Anonymous meetings with your family and attending Gam-Anon meetings.

CONCLUSIONS

Because pathological gamblers can no longer control their gambling, their gambling activities become the main priority in their lives over their responsibilities to self and family. As a result, the pathological gambler, spouse or partner, and children are likely to experience mental disorders, health problems related to stress, substance abuse and addiction, financial strain, and legal problems. The children are the most victimized of all in this situation as they are robbed of developing in a healthy family environment that can serve as a model for their future families.

However, there is help for families in which there is a pathological gambler. Support groups and professional therapists use a family approach to help gamblers overcome and cope with their negative behavior and family issues.

See also: Gender and Gambling; Peer Pressure and Gambling; School and Work Performance and Gambling; Youth at Special Risk

FURTHER READING
Kalischuk, R. "Cocreating Life Pathways: Problem Gambling and Its Impact on Families." *The Family Journal* 18, no. 1 (2010).

■ GAMBLING, HISTORY OF

The evolution of the phenomenon or behavior in which a person chooses risk over a certain outcome. Gambling is thought to be older than humanity. In fact, scientists have found evidence of gambling behavior in animals, situations in which animals chose risk over certainty when performing a task for a reward. Games of chance have been discovered in the earliest human societies. Although gambling has evolved and flourished throughout human development, each new derivation contains basic elements from the phenomenon's origins. From knucklebones to big casinos, gambling has undergone many changes throughout its long history.

THE BIRTH OF GAMBLING

Remnants of gambling can be traced back to the Paleolithic era. During this time, astragali, or animal anklebones, were used in a way similar to that of modern-day dice. Today, we refer to the astragali dice as knucklebones, a name probably derived from a game in which one places astragali on one's knuckles, turns his or her hand, and tries to catch the bones before they fall. The knucklebones have been found throughout Mesopotamia, the location thought to be the site where modern civilization began to form. In fact, the bones were found consistently through each phase of Mesopotamian history. In a site dated to 3000 B.C., the earliest form of modern-day dice was found, the bones shaven with markings on each side.

Gambling, therefore, began with knucklebones. Early on, knucklebones were used for religious activities or telling the future, but as time wore on, they were used instead for entertainment. Rolling the knucklebones became a game of chance, one where wagers could be made.

Gambling is even incorporated into Greek mythology. Casting lots decided where Zeus, Poseidon, and Hades would reign. The results of the throw sent Zeus to the heavens, Poseidon to the sea, and Hades to the underworld. The Greeks themselves introduced a new kind of gambling in the fifth century B.C. in the form of cock fighting.

The Roman Empire adopted the Greek traditions of cock fighting and dicing and added another form of gambling—wagering on games of skill. History shows that the Romans began placing bets on stadium games such as chariot races. The Roman emperors thoroughly enjoyed gambling: Emperors Augustus, Caligula, and Claudius gambled with fervor despite laws passed to minimize this activity. Roman officials attempted to limit the incidence of gambling by fining perpetrators with fees four times the wager and prohibiting people from suing for their payments.

Romans were not the only society to pass laws in an effort to restrict or prohibit gambling. Christian, Jewish, and Islamic religious leaders also wrote or campaigned for laws to prohibit gambling in their societies. Although the New Testament, or Christian Bible, mentions lot casting throughout the text, both Christians and Jews generally frowned on gambling. Islam was the first religion to outlaw gambling in any form. Followers of Islam believed that gambling and consuming alcohol were the handiwork of the devil.

Gambling also was prohibited throughout medieval Europe. Still, although it was expressly prohibited, gambling was prevalent throughout Europe in the forms of using knucklebones similar to jacks or marbles, cock fighting, and wagering on public games. Literature of the time documented the pervasiveness of gambling, as in Geoffrey Chaucer's *Canterbury Tales*.

THE MODERNIZATION OF GAMBLING

Around the second millennium A.D., playing cards emerged and are thought to have originated in Korea. The first Korean card decks contained 80 cards, which consisted of eight suits with 10 cards in each suit. These cards were rectangular and roughly eight inches in length by two inches in width. China developed the next batch of playing cards, which seem to be the antecedents of modern playing cards. These decks contained 52 cards with four different suits. The pictures on the Chinese cards were illustrated in black or red and were depicted as mirror images, so that the player was able to read the card no matter the direction in which it was held.

The playing cards used today emerged around 1870 A.D., after many years of development and the input of several different cultures. As cards became more prevalent in gambling, lawmakers began to rewrite existing laws to prohibit placing wagers on card games. Also, in Italy, church officials took a strong stance against gambling and demonstrated the position of the Catholic Church by conducting mass burnings of gambling materials.

Around 1444, **lotteries** emerged in Europe. The original lottery was put in place to raise funds for improvements in Rome. This lottery used a draw method similar to the powerballs of today. Lotteries spread like wildfire throughout Europe, encountering only mild occasional opposition. The 16th century sparked a revolution in gambling: the **science of probability** was discovered. This breakthrough in understanding odds allowed people to apply mathematical principles to gambling. Players had more control in the game and were able to manipulate their outcomes in ways they were unable to before. The 16th century also brought about the birth of public gambling houses, the predecessor to casinos. The gambling houses remained open until the 1700s, when lawmakers brought about a new wave of prohibition laws.

GAMBLING IN AMERICA

American gambling is a fusion of customs from Native American, African, and European cultures. Historically, Native Americans took gambling seriously. Certain games were played in accordance with what people believed the gods wanted. Although much of the gambling was performed as a style of fortune-telling, many Native Americans also used gambling as a means to redistribute goods throughout the community. The English settlers brought European gambling to America. The game of choice became horse racing, and by 1700, there were 12 horse tracks throughout the New England colonies. Horse racing and card games remained the most popular forms of gambling until 1793, when the first American lottery was established. In fact, this lottery was created to help finance the construction of Washington, D.C. Lotteries gained instant popularity and were used as ways to improve and build cities in America.

As lotteries boomed, so did scam artists. The surge of scam artists pretending to sell lottery chances and then leaving with the collected money led the state legislatures to look more carefully at the lotteries. Although lotteries waxed and waned over many years, they today remain popular in many states.

In the late 1850s, many Americans traveled west to seek gold in the California gold rush. California banned gaming houses but allowed social gambling. As a result, people looked toward Nevada to fulfill their gambling needs. The territorial governor of Nevada outlawed gambling from the start. When Nevada became a state in 1864, the legislature began pushing for the legalization of gambling. The supporters of gambling achieved their goal in 1869 when gambling was decriminalized in Nevada. Reno, Nevada became the premier gambling hot spot. Large gambling clubs and casinos became popular, and slot machines began to fill restaurants and stores. Gambling gained momentum and started to sprout up in towns throughout Nevada. One such town was Las Vegas, known for its strip of grandiose casinos. Las Vegas was established during the Great Depression as a way to stimulate the tanking economy. The city has evolved into a multibillion-dollar tourist attraction.

Gambling today

American gambling evolved quickly over the next few decades, resulting in changes in laws and legalization in most states. Currently, gambling is legal in all states except Utah and Hawaii, and casinos can operate in 27 states. Many legal gambling venues are located on Native American reservations. In the late 1970s, lawsuits were filed on the issues of state control over Native American land. Rulings dictated that state government had no jurisdiction over the Native American reservations. The Supreme Court case of *California v. Cabazon Band of Mission Indians* ruled that state government could not prohibit gaming on reservation land. Other legal gambling venues consist of riverboats and online games.

Despite its long history, gambling still inspires controversy. Although gambling is legal in many countries, the types of gambling that are legal vary from country to country and state to state. Overall, legal gambling has caused lawmakers to reconsider their rules and regulations because of the detrimental effect frequent gambling has on the lives of those who participate.

See also: Law and Gambling, The

FURTHER READING
Dunstan, R. *Gambling in California.* Sacramento: California Research Bureau, 1997.
Schwartz, David G. *Roll the Bones: The History of Gambling.* New York: Gotham Books, 2006.

▓ GENDER AND GAMBLING

The biological and behavioral differences between males and females and the effect of those differences on gambling. Most research has been focused on the male experience of gambling. This may be due to several factors. First, in many countries, men were allowed to gamble legally for decades before women. Secondly, gambling has a negative stigma, which may result in women's seeking treatment for gambling problems at lower rates than men, even though, in general, women seek counseling for mental health issues more often than men. Last, most of the treatment programs created do not meet the needs of women.

Also, studies have found that men and women differ in their choice of games. Whereas men tend to choose gaming that is action-oriented, such as poker, which requires high-risk wagers, women are drawn to gambling that offers escape, such as slot machines, which require low risk and low social interaction.

Fact Or Fiction?

Women do not spend as much money on gambling as men.

The Facts: Research has shown that, on average, women do not spend as much money on gambling as men do. Most women who gamble play video poker, slot machines, or lotteries. Due to the nature of these games, women would need to spend substantially more time in the act of gambling to spend as much money as those who play high-stake games like

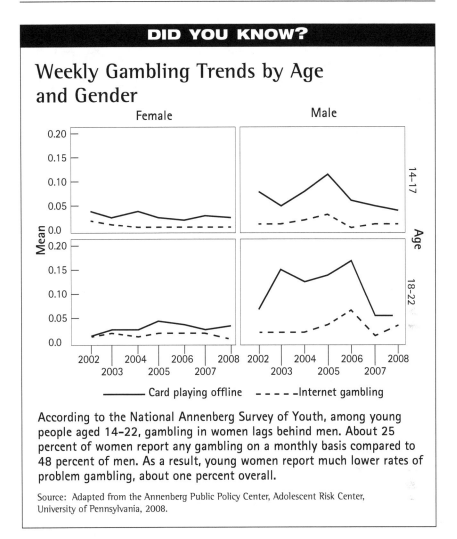

DID YOU KNOW?

Weekly Gambling Trends by Age and Gender

Female   Male

—— Card playing offline   - - - - Internet gambling

According to the National Annenberg Survey of Youth, among young people aged 14-22, gambling in women lags behind men. About 25 percent of women report any gambling on a monthly basis compared to 48 percent of men. As a result, young women report much lower rates of problem gambling, about one percent overall.

Source: Adapted from the Annenberg Public Policy Center, Adolescent Risk Center, University of Pennsylvania, 2008.

poker, blackjack, and craps. Although statistically women do not spend or risk as much money as men, low-stake gambling still results in debt and in both family and legal problems.

Although demographic data does indicate that men gamble more than women, the incidence of women's gambling is rising exponentially. The prevalence of male versus female gamblers may be due to under-reporting, which in turn is due to the stigmatizing label of *gambler*.

GENDER AND TREATMENT

Research also has shown that women are more likely to seek mental health treatment as compared to men. The dissonance between women's seeking treatment and the lack of women involved in treatment programs for gambling is considered to be the result of several factors. Due to the predominately male presence in the research on gambling, many treatment programs were designed specifically for men. Because male-dominated groups can be intimidating, for example, women may not feel comfortable disclosing information. Also, even if a woman does seek mental health treatment, she most likely will not be screened for a gambling problem. Additionally, because most treatment programs were designed for men, staff may not be adequately trained to work with female gamblers. Among other drawbacks, treatment programs may not have child care.

GENDER SOCIALIZATION AND GAMBLING

Games attract the genders differently. Because boys and girls are reared differently, men are known for being "action gamblers," and women are known for being "escape gamblers." An action gambler has a need for high risks and high stakes. This type of gambling involves table games such as poker and blackjack. An action gambler seeks games that are charged with energy and anxiety. These gamblers tend to be Type A males. A Type A personality is characterized by impatience, urgency, and competitiveness. Typically, action gamblers begin gambling at an early age, usually during adolescence, when underage gambling is illegal. Although action gamblers appear to be confident and assertive, they often have low self-esteem. Gambling becomes an outlet for people to feel as though they are raising their self-esteem. Although action gamblers favor skill-based games and high-risk stakes, they lose more than they win. Although this group is primarily male, many women also fit into this category.

Most women for whom gambling is a compulsion can be labeled escape gamblers, although many men also gamble for escape. These gamblers favor games of pure chance like playing slot machines and lotteries. These individuals use gambling to escape the stresses of their lives.

Escape gambling tends to occur later in life, anywhere between the ages of 30 and 80. Many of these individuals have experienced childhood abuse or a crisis or loss of some sort. For example, another reason women begin to gamble may be a result of the Empty Nest

Syndrome, whose children have moved away from home, a type of loss. Parents, particularly women, may become lonely and depressed. These parents may visit casinos to pass the time and, as a result, dull their feelings of loneliness through the excitement of gambling.

WHO PLAYS WHAT AND WHEN

Men and women gamble differently and with different games. Women tend to begin gambling later in life, and most often women use gambling as a way to escape problems. Men tend to gamble with high stakes in hands-on, action-oriented games. They tend to begin gambling early in life, usually during adolescence. Most gambling begins socially and as a way to achieve an **adrenaline** rush. After time, individuals who seek the rush build up a tolerance to its effect; they feel a need to gamble more and more and are said to suffer from a behavioral addiction. The nature of action games is high-stake, which often results in big losses and the individual's chasing the loss, or gambling more despite a negative outcome. Although most treatments are designed for the male gambler, treatment is available for both genders.

TEENS SPEAK

The Rush Pulled Me In

My name is Amber and I'm 17 years old. I got into gambling recently. My parents are getting a divorce, and I've been feeling really alone. My parents think I'm old enough to understand their situation, and my friends don't really get how I feel. There's really no one I can talk to. I started gambling on a quest to find something to take my mind off the divorce. I don't do drugs and I don't drink but I've spent a lot of time sitting around feeling depressed. I couldn't handle the pain and my grades started to drop. One day, I went into the local convenience store, where they have a bunch of slot machines.

At first the rush pulled me in. I wasn't supposed to be gambling, but no one noticed me. I guess it was a rebellion at first; maybe I wanted my parents to pay attention to me. Pretty quickly, playing the slot machines made me forget about my problems. Alone with myself, there were no questions and no sympathetic looks. I won sometimes but was afraid to cash out my tickets because the staff would find out I was underage.

Anytime I felt down or got bad grades, I would think about going to the store. I started lying to my friends and parents. After a while, I found myself ditching class to go play; I started spending all of my paycheck from my part-time job, not because I was losing, but because I would spend about 12 hours per day at my machine. I got to know the other regulars; it was like a family.

I had created so many lies that by the time I realized I had a problem, I had no one to ask for help. What would they think of me? I didn't want to get in trouble.

Eventually, I told my mom how I was feeling, although I didn't admit to gambling. She sent me to a counselor, and I told her about my gambling. I thought gambling helped me escape from my feelings, but the funny thing was that my feelings were still there when I wasn't gambling. I wasted half a year only to find myself in the same place emotionally. My counselor suggested I attend Gamblers Anonymous meetings. I understand more about myself now and feel lucky I was able to recover relatively unharmed.

See also: Adolescents and Gambling; Social Gambling

FURTHER READING

Matheson, Kimberly, Michael J. A. Wohl, and Hymie Anisman. "The Interplay of Appraisals, Specific Coping Styles, and Depressive Symptoms Among Young Male and Female Gamblers." *Social Psychology* (2009).

Stevens, Matthew, and Martin Young. "Who Plays What? Participation Profiles in Chance Versus Skill-based Gambling." *Journal of Gambling Studies* (2010).

▤ HELP FOR GAMBLERS

Getting treatment for those who repeatedly play games of chance for money or something of value. Gambling can be as addictive as drugs such as crack/cocaine. The activity changes brain chemistry just like any other addictive psychoactive substances. Problem gambling occurs in roughly 1 to 2 percent of the population. Treatment for problem gambling focuses on the addiction and aims to rehabilitate the gambler. In treatment, problem gamblers undergo counseling and **rehabilitation** as well as attend self-help groups. The most common form of help for gamblers is Gamblers Anonymous. Other forms of treatment consist of counseling by using cognitive behavioral therapy and inpatient and outpatient rehabilitation.

GAMBLERS ANONYMOUS

Gambling is a newly recognized addiction, and treatment options are continuously evolving. The most popular treatment for problem gamblers is Gamblers Anonymous. The organization was the idea of two men who decided to meet and discuss their problems with gambling and the devastating effects it had on their lives. They began to meet every week, and, after a few meetings, the men realized they had ceased gambling. Their meetings were so helpful that they decided to create an official group. The first official meeting of Gamblers Anonymous occurred on Friday, September 13, 1957. Gamblers Anonymous grew quickly and continues to grow and evolve today.

Gamblers Anonymous follows the standard twelve-step protocol that is used in groups like Alcoholics Anonymous (AA) and Narcotics Anonymous (NA). Each Gamblers Anonymous meeting lasts about one and a half to two hours, which is longer than AA and NA meetings. Because problem gambling is a newly recognized addiction, locations housing Gamblers Anonymous meetings are not widespread. If a town does not have easy access to Gamblers Anonymous meetings, help can be found through attending AA or NA meetings where a counselor may be able to direct the problem gambler to those who specialize in the treatment of problem gambling.

Gamblers Anonymous provides a special service to new members, Pressure Relief Groups. These groups are open to new members who have maintained 30 to 60 days of **abstinence** and have attended at least three meetings. Pressure Relief Groups provide counseling to the gambler and his or her partner for issues surrounding debt, employment, and family concerns or conflicts. Much like AA, Gamblers Anonymous has a sister group devoted to helping the families of the gamblers. Gam-Anon is the equivalent of Al-Anon, a group specifically for the families and friends of alcoholics. Similarly, Gam-Anon serves the family and friends of the problem gambler. Gam-Anon meets once a month with Gamblers Anonymous to discuss pertinent issues and facilitate camaraderie between the gambler and the family.

TREATMENT AND REHABILITATION

Research has found cognitive behavioral therapy to be an effective therapy for problem gambling. Cognitive behavioral therapy is a structured therapy that focuses on changing thoughts and behaviors. It can be used in both group and individual counseling settings. **Group therapy** that uses cognitive behavioral therapy works well for problem gamblers, because it allows the members to learn from each other and is cost effective. Cognitive behavioral therapy also works well with other forms of therapy and **twelve-step programs** like Gamblers Anonymous.

Gambling treatment and rehabilitation is practiced in residential, inpatient, and intensive outpatient settings. Residential and inpatient settings are very similar in that individuals live on site for treatment. Each facility is staffed 24 hours per day to provide extensive rehabilitation to each gambler. Residential facilities concentrate on behavioral disorders and mental illness. These facilities can be freestanding or located in a hospital setting, and the length of care is usually longer than in inpatient settings. Inpatient care uses a bio-psycho-social model of care, in which problem gamblers are provided a therapeutic, protective environment that offers comprehensive medical and psychiatric help. An individual's length of stay in an inpatient setting should depend on that person's level of addiction and rate of progress in the treatment. Many inpatient facilities offer aftercare in the form of outpatient care, which can be intensive. Residential and inpatient care may not be convenient or possible for some individuals seeking treatment. Many people cannot leave their jobs or family for extended periods of time or do not have any or sufficient insurance coverage for treatment.

Fact Or Fiction?

Las Vegas, Nevada, and Atlantic City, New Jersey are the only locations that have counselors who specialize in gambling addiction.

The Facts: Gambling is legal in all but two states, Utah and Hawaii. Although gambling is illegal in those states, individuals can still access online gambling, the stock market, and lotteries. While life in Las Vegas and Atlantic City is centered around gambling, people in all 50 states have easy access to gambling. Wherever gambling exists, so will addiction, as will counselors who specialize in treating behavioral addictions. In fact, the National Council on Problem Gambling has affiliates in most states. If your state does not have an affiliate, the Council will locate a nationally certified gambling counselor in your area. See "Hotlines and Help Sites" at the back of this book for detailed information.

Intensive outpatient care offers individuals convenient hours for intense therapy. In an intensive outpatient program, individuals come in three to five days per week for several hours of individual and group counseling. Most locations offer these services during both evening and daytime hours so that the individuals seeking treatment can attend to their families and employment while getting better. Outpatient care is similar to individual counseling. In this setting, the gambler can expect to devote a few hours per week to individual and group counseling.

There are many outlets worldwide for the treatment of problem gambling. Gambling is a real addiction and can be life-altering. Admitting there is a problem is scary and seeking help can be an intimidating task. There is treatment available regardless of a person's level of gambling, financial background, or ability to devote time. Gamblers Anonymous, counseling, and rehabilitation centers are reliable options for treatment.

TEENS SPEAK

I Was a Problem Gambler

I started gambling with my friends when I was 12. It was fun and at first we didn't use money. We would bet things like food or our skateboards or CDs. It got boring quickly so we started to bet small amounts of money. We were kids, so it didn't seem dangerous. I always watched my dad play poker with his buddies or bet on football. Gambling made me feel like a grownup.

When I entered high school, my gambling became intense. I got a part-time job to help out at home and to have money to go to the movies, shop, or just grab some food. Instead of helping out or going out to the movies, however, I ended up playing games like poker with my friends and betting on football with my dad. It felt exhilarating and I loved to win. I spent all day thinking about it. I couldn't concentrate in class on the days I knew I would be playing games with my buddies. I'd fantasize about how I'd spend the money, maybe help my parents buy a new dishwasher or get a new video game. Instead of winning, I'd often lose all of my paycheck. Once I started playing, I couldn't stop. I'd win one hand and get greedy; then I'd lose and get scared. I spent most of my time trying to win back the money I'd lost. My friends always invited me to play; I didn't realize that it was because they knew I'd always end up playing until I had nothing.

I didn't realize my gambling was a problem until my mom caught me stealing money from her purse. I broke her trust, but in my mind, I just wanted to win my money back. She thought I was using the money for drugs and brought me to a therapist. I didn't think I had a problem. I spent a few months in therapy and realized that what I was going through was a real addiction. I felt depressed and ashamed. I had stolen several times from my mom and my job. My therapist helped me work on myself and rebuild relationships I had lost through gambling. I started going to a group called Gamblers Anonymous. It was surprising and reassuring to see that other people had the same problem.

Since starting therapy and going to Gamblers Anonymous, I have made amends with my parents and started paying back my debts. Because my grades dropped when I was gambling, I've been working hard to raise them back up. As for my friends, they know about my problems with gambling and now don't invite me over to play poker. I am appreciative that they respect my recovery but wonder if anyone else in our group is going through the same thing. Getting treatment for my gambling was the best thing that could have happened for me. I turned my life around. If I could go back in time, I would not have started gambling.

It's addictive and can take control of your life before you even realize it.

See also: Prevention and Intervention; Protective Factors

FURTHER READING
Sojourner, M. *She Bets Her Life: A True Story of Gambling Addiction.* Berkeley, Calif.: Seal Press, 2010.

■ INTERNET AND ONLINE GAMBLING, THE

As of 2010, it was estimated that almost 2 billion people worldwide were using the Internet, and Internet, or online, gambling is the fastest growing segment of the gaming industry. The first site for Internet gambling was created in 1995. In 1997, approximately 30 gambling Web sites were available, but by 2007, that number had grown to an estimated 3,000 gambling Web sites. In the United States, the gambling age at most online casinos is 18.

AVAILABILITY TO TEENS

Adolescents have easy access to the Internet through schools, public libraries, Internet cafes, and home computers. With ready access, and given that teens spend a great deal of unsupervised time online, they are especially vulnerable for problem gambling. In fact, current studies show that one in five Internet gamblers, which include young adult gamblers, have a pathological gambling problem.

Additionally, online gambling is particularly appealing to teens, for whom it is illegal to gamble, because the user is anonymous, parental approval is unnecessary, and site operators enforce few restrictions. As a result, there is ample opportunity for those who are underage (in online gambling, anyone under 18) to gamble.

LEGALIZATION OF INTERNET GAMBLING

The legalization of Internet gambling is a hotly contested issue. Opponents of legalized online gambling argue that Internet gambling will lead to an increase in the negative personal and public issues that surround problem and pathological gambling. Proponents of online gambling support the increased tax revenues that would be collected through legalization. Advocates for online poker, for example, are particularly opposed to a gambling ban; they maintain that poker is a game of skill rather than chance. Because of its popularity and the difficulty in regulating the game, revenue from online poker is between 34 million and 200 million dollars every month. Others advocate for an environment where Internet gambling is regulated and taxed by the federal government. Currently, online gambling revenue in the United States is estimated at between 7 and 10 billion dollars a year and is expected to reach more than 24 billion dollars in 2010.

The current law
In October 2006, the U.S. government passed the Unlawful Internet Gambling Enforcement Act (UIGEA) to combat online gambling, which is illegal. However, the lack of serious enforcement makes it extremely difficult to accomplish all of the law's objectives. Another obstacle to enforcing this law is a loose definition of what is unlawful.

Currently, 51 members of the U.S. House of Representatives are working to pass legislation that will regulate Internet gambling while protecting the consumer. Legal arguments attempting to classify poker as a game of skill have failed. In *People v. Mitchell,* the Illinois Appellate Court upheld a jury's conclusion that a skill-based exception did not apply to poker games. Likewise, the Colorado Supreme Court found in *Chames v. Central City Opera House Association* that poker constitutes "a form of 'gambling' in its commonly understood sense" because it in fact relies on elements of chance. As a result, many Internet gambling companies have pulled out of the U.S. market for fear of being prosecuted by the U.S. Department of Justice.

WHAT MAKES ONLINE POKER POPULAR?
Online poker's popularity boom was caused by the explosion of televised live poker on numerous national networks. Major poker events, such as The World Series of Poker, offer millions of dollars in prizes, but the entry fees are very high. As a result, a large number of Internet gamblers play online poker for a chance to gain free entry into televised events. In the 2003 World Series of Poker, for example, "everyman" Chris Moneymaker won his entry to the event through an online qualification. Also, with downloadable poker programs being offered through the Internet, both experienced and novice gamblers—as well as underage gamblers—were able to play. In one 2005 estimate, it was found that nearly 100,000 people were playing

online poker for money during peak hours of the day, and almost an equal number were participating in free games.

NEGATIVE IMPACTS OF INTERNET GAMING

In one study, researchers ranked legalized gambling as the third leading cause of individual bankruptcies in the United States. The study also found credit card use to be a critical link between bankruptcy and gambling. Because almost all Internet gambling is facilitated either directly or indirectly through credit card charges, the legalization of online gambling would likely increase a person's financial debt.

Young adults are especially vulnerable

Unfortunately, the lack of age verification on Internet gaming sites allows teenagers to gamble online.

Young adults, especially college students, are a vulnerable group because they often possess or have access to credit cards with no parental supervision. These individuals tend to be unaware of the consequences of abusing and mismanaging credit, while also lacking the **impulse control** necessary to handle addictive behaviors, including gambling. Among the common harms experienced by pathological Internet gamblers are

- emotional distress associated with gambling losses (100 percent)
- financial problems (85.7 percent)
- insomnia (57.1 percent)
- poor physical health (42.9 percent)
- weakened academic performance (42.9 percent)
- damaged family relationships (28.6 percent)
- disrupted part-time work (14.3 percent)

INTERNET GAMBLING AND PROBLEM GAMBLING

Because of the public's fear that gambling is accompanied by problem behaviors and criminal activity, the popularity of Internet gambling has caused much concern and debate. Current studies have found that the immediate gratification and high level of privacy afforded by the lax rules and anonymity of the Internet can indeed increase the occurrence of problem gaming. This result is not surprising considering the speed at which online gaming and money wagers take place.

For example, rather than playing about 30 hands per hour at a live game, a poker player can average 60 to 80 hands per hour online. In other words, with fast-paced Internet gambling, there is greater financial loss. In fact, Internet gamblers wager 8.5 more times per bet than casino gamblers. Researchers also suggest that the potential for problem gambling is higher among online participants than on-site gamblers. They estimate that the rate of problem gambling among Internet gamblers is 10 times higher than the rate among the general population. Studies reveal

- 35.7 percent of Internet gamblers can be classified as excessive online gamblers who have experienced harm brought about by their activity.
- In one North American study, 43 percent of the gamblers interviewed met the criteria for either moderate or severe problem gambling.

ONLINE GAMBLING AND MENTAL HEALTH

In other articles in this book, it is clear that pathological gambling, regardless of its form, is associated with financial difficulties, emotional distress, and psychiatric problems, such as mood disorders like **bipolar disorder**. However, of additional and growing concern is that Internet gambling, a sedentary and isolating activity, may place one at risk for other mental health problems. In one survey of more than 43,000 respondents, pathological gambling was associated with increased odds of every psychiatric disorder assessed.

See also: Adolescents and Gambling; Risk Taking and Gambling; Types of Gambling

FURTHER READING

Haddock, Patricia. *Teens and Gambling: Who Wins?* Berkeley Heights, N.J.: Enslow Publishers, 1996.

North American Training Institute. *Wanna Bet? Everything You Wanted to Know About Teen Gambling but Never Thought to Ask.* Duluth, Minn.: North American Training Institute, 1997.

Petry, N. M., and J. Weinstock. "Internet Gambling Is Common in College Students and Associated with Poor Mental Health." *The American Journal on Addictions* 16 (2007).

■ INTERVENTION
See: Prevention and Intervention

■ LAW AND GAMBLING, THE
The statutes or rules that govern gaming and gaming behaviors. Underlying all reasoned laws is public policy, that is, the reasons that government is attempting to achieve certain goals by adopting a law. Public policy can be based on many considerations: moral, political, health, safety, social, and economic. Once a government sets policy goals, it must adopt specific laws to meet them. Violations of these laws can result in either civil or criminal sanctions or a combination of both.

GAMING LAWS
Laws are rules that a society establishes to govern its conduct; gaming laws are the rules established to govern the conduct of gaming. Gaming control involves the adoption, interpretation, and enforcement of laws that dictate how or whether persons may offer or participate in gambling transactions. Every industrialized country has some form of gaming law, even countries or states that prohibit it. Some governments impose severe punishments for gambling infractions, while others levy light penalties. These laws and their enforcement reflect how gambling is conducted.

GAMBLING ADDICTION AND ADOLESCENTS
While the majority of adults who gamble do so responsibly and, therefore, do not experience any gambling-related problems, gambling can be a powerful form of addiction for many individuals, including adolescents. In fact, some researchers have concluded that adolescents are about three times more likely than adults to become problem gamblers. Beyond the huge debt and financial difficulties frequently experienced by gamblers, both problem and pathological gambling have been linked to a host of additional negative consequences, including, but not limited to, increased domestic violence, substance use disorders, crime, suicide, and the deterioration of both physical and mental health.

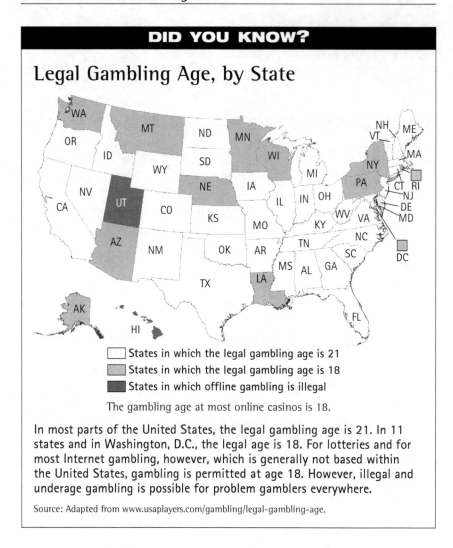

DID YOU KNOW?

Legal Gambling Age, by State

☐ States in which the legal gambling age is 21
▨ States in which the legal gambling age is 18
■ States in which offline gambling is illegal

The gambling age at most online casinos is 18.

In most parts of the United States, the legal gambling age is 21. In 11 states and in Washington, D.C., the legal age is 18. For lotteries and for most Internet gambling, however, which is generally not based within the United States, gambling is permitted at age 18. However, illegal and underage gambling is possible for problem gamblers everywhere.

Source: Adapted from www.usaplayers.com/gambling/legal-gambling-age.

These gambling-related problems take a toll on both individuals and society as a whole. As a result, the consequences of problem and pathological gambling raise important questions about the responsibility of government to educate the public.

THE CONTROVERSY OVER GAMBLING IN THE UNITED STATES

The words *gambling* and *gaming* are used interchangeably to describe an activity in which something of value is risked on the chance that something of greater value might be obtained, based on the uncertain outcome of a particular event. The word *gaming,* which can be traced to *gamen,* the Old English word for "game," once described betting on games such as cards and dice. Later, in the late 18th century, opponents of gaming coined the term *gambling,* a term that was developed to indicate their disapproval and stigmatize the activity.

The use of two different words to describe the same activity reflects the long-standing controversy over legalized gambling in the United States. Throughout the nation's history, Americans have either fought for or contested the right to wager, or place a bet. Advocates for gambling have heralded it as a savior of state economies, while opponents have decried it as a moral demon. As a result of the ambiguous attitude toward gambling, gambling activities in America have been alternately condemned, banned, tolerated, legalized, and regulated throughout the course of the country's history.

The early days

Gambling in North America preceded the foundation of the United States. Arriving on the Atlantic seaboard in the 16th and 17th centuries, European settlers and explorers encountered native tribes that had well-established systems of wagering. For example, early explorers in New York witnessed members of the Onondaga tribe placing bets on the roll of stone dice.

While such gambling was a form of recreation for American Indians, it also contained a religious dimension. In fact, for most native tribes, casting dice or engaging in other games of chance was a method used for divining the favor of the gods.

In the early days of the republic, the banking system was primitive and the government imposed few taxes. As a result, public officials turned to **lotteries** to pay for necessary public works projects such as the building of roads, bridges, and canals. Lotteries also raised funds for the Continental Army during the Revolutionary War and were responsible, in part, for financing the development of the District of Columbia and some of the first American universities, such as Harvard, Yale, Columbia, and Dartmouth.

Still, many colonists had strong moral objections to gambling. For example, the Puritans, who settled much of New England, opposed gambling because they believed that it undermined the "Protestant ethic" of self-control, hard work, and thrift. Many religious leaders also condemned gambling, because they believed that it destroyed families and communities and exposed gamblers to other vices such as alcohol and prostitution. In fact, opposition to gambling was so strong in the 17th century that Massachusetts lawmakers passed laws prohibiting not only card playing and dice but also shuffleboard and bowling.

PUBLIC POLICIES

In general, a society's public policy regarding gaming usually falls into one of four categories. The least restrictive policy treats gambling as an acceptable activity in which its citizens and residents may participate without government interference. The most restrictive policy views gambling as an undesirable activity that government should not tolerate. The viewpoint lying between these two polar opposites views gambling, whether legal or not, as an inevitable activity. Consequently, proponents of the middle-of-the-road view think that government should permit gambling, but they should permit it in such a manner that it is not encouraged. The fourth common policy position allows gambling if its benefits outweigh its burdens. In all cases, theological, philosophical, social, and economic arguments are offered in order to support or decry each public policy position. Clearly, the legalization and regulation of commercial gambling involves a wide range of issues.

The policy of restriction

A review of the history of gambling shows that prohibition, in which gambling is an undesirable activity, has generally failed to eliminate gambling for a number of reasons. First, gambling has been and continues to be a popular and inevitable human activity irrespective of laws. In *The Business of Risk,* Vicki Abt and her coauthors observed that "gambling is a universal cultural phenomenon: one of a relatively small number of activities that occur in nearly all societies and every period. People have been playing risky games for at least 4,000 years, and virtually every culture has evolved ways of letting its members stake something of value on an event of uncertain outcome."

Secondly, prohibition often results in unintended negative consequences. In fact, many people believe that laws against gambling may lead to even worse consequences than gaming itself. For example, some argue that prohibition only serves to drive gambling "underground," into the hands of organized crime, where gaming syndicates have a monopoly on power, governments collect no tax revenues, and victims of cheating have no legal recourse.

Sports betting provides a modern-day example of why prohibition does not work. Even though many forms of gaming are widely available, betting on sports is legal in only one state, Nevada. Nonetheless, the National Gambling Impact Study Commission (NGISC) called sports betting the most widespread and popular form of gaming in America, with an estimated $80 billion to $380 billion wagered every year. In 2006, only a tiny percentage of that amount—$2.43 billion—was wagered legally. Authorities believe that the balance is handled by organized crime.

Thirdly, gaming prohibition raises the question of government's role with respect to gambling itself. Many individuals challenge the legitimacy of government's interference with citizens' private lives. They question whether or not the government has the right to tell adults how to spend their money or to punish people for engaging in behavior that does not directly harm others. A basic tenet of democracy asserts that people who live in a free society have the right to live the way they choose.

GOVERNMENT'S INTEREST IN GAMBLING

The formulation of public policy on gambling is further complicated by the fact that government has an economic interest in gambling. In fact, when governments discover gambling as a source of public revenue, they develop an interest in promoting it. For example, much of the motivation for the growth of legalized gambling in 20th-century America resulted from state governments' need to increase revenue.

State revenues

Since 1964, when New Hampshire created the first lottery of the 20th century, state governments have embraced lotteries as a source of revenue in lieu of more conventional forms of taxation. Described as "painless" or "voluntary" taxes, lotteries are much easier for politicians to propose and implement than other taxation alternatives. At the beginning of 2005, 39 states plus the District of Columbia were operating lotteries, and total lottery sales were a little more than $34 billion. Also, on average, states retained approximately half of the money that was wagered.

LEGALIZATION AND PROBLEM GAMBLING

Clearly, state governments have seen significant revenue benefits from the legalization of commercial gambling. However, research makes it equally clear that one of the major costs associated with the expansion of legalized gambling is the increase of problem and pathological gambling.

The results from a number of studies reveal that 1.2 percent to 1.6 percent of the adult North American population can be considered pathological gamblers, while an additional 1.5 percent are problem gamblers, and another 7.7 percent are identified as "at risk" of becoming problem gamblers. Although the prevalence of pathological and problem gambling cannot be attributed solely to the legalization of gambling, legalization has made it easier for gamblers to access gambling venues. It has also created "new" gamblers, individuals who might not have considered gambling in illegal or unpleasant circumstances (for example, numbers parlors operated by organized crime, race tracks, casinos).

GOVERNMENT RESPONSIBILITY

In light of the fact that states receive substantial revenues from lotteries and from taxes imposed on other gambling venues, do they, in turn, have a responsibility to spend some of those revenues on developing programs that educate the public about problem and pathological gambling, developing prevention programs, and providing treatment services for problem and pathological gamblers?

Currently, there is no national policy on problem gambling, and most states have made little funding available for problem gambling, especially compared to the funds outlaid for substance-abuse programs. The legal gambling opportunities created by states in the 1980s and 1990s are not going to disappear, and they may actually increase. Having created these opportunities, the next step is for state policy makers to address the negative consequences of problem and pathological gambling.

See also: Addiction and Gambling; Crime and Gambling; Gambling, History of; Public Health Issues and Gambling

FURTHER READING

Evans, Rod, and Mark Hance, eds. *Legalized Gambling: For and Against.* Peru, Ill.: Open Court Publishing Company, 1998.

Haugen, David. *Library in a Book: Legalized Gambling.* New York: Infobase Publishing, 2006.

Ruschmann, Paul. *Legalized Gambling.* New York: Chelsea House, 2009.

University of Nevada Las Vegas, International Gaming Institute. *The Gaming Industry: Introduction and Perspectives.* Hoboken, N.J.: John Wiley & Sons, Inc., 1996.

■ MONEY PROBLEMS AND GAMBLING

See: Crime and Gambling

■ ONLINE GAMBLING

See: Internet and Online Gambling, The

■ PEER PRESSURE AND GAMBLING

The strong influence that a particular social group has on the attitudes and behaviors of each of its individual members and the effect of that influence on a person's risk-taking behavior, such as gambling. Peer pressure is strongest during adolescence and comes from other individuals with whom teenagers identify.

Pressure on a person occurs when his or her peer group persuades or coerces the individual to adopt similar values, goals, and beliefs and to participate in the group's activities. Peer pressure can have either positive or negative influences.

POSITIVE AND NEGATIVE PEER PRESSURE AND GAMBLING

Usually associated with negative influences, peer pressure can impact an individual's substance use, bullying, vandalism, gossiping, stealing, or cutting class. However, there are other social groups whose activities or attitudes have positive influences on their members. For example, after-school organizations and clubs that can have a positive impact might include science club, computer club, the debate team, or organized sports activities. The extent of influence a group has on a member depends a great deal on an adolescent's family values and upbringing.

FAMILY INFLUENCE AND RISK FACTORS

Beginning about age three, children attempt to copy the behavior of the adults around them. Children surrounded with positive adult role models and peer friendships during this critical developmental period tend to be less influenced by negative peer pressure during their adolescence. In fact, family behaviors and attitudes toward gambling, alcohol, tobacco, and illegal substances can help prepare a teen to make the appropriate choices when faced with both negative and positive peer pressure.

Family values and exposure to positive and negative influences also can have a long-term effect on young people, one that will continue into their adult lives. For example, a lack of parental supervision coupled with peer pressure can be relevant factors in gambling behavior. In fact, the biggest influence on teenage gambling is having parents who gamble. Research studies show higher rates of problem gambling among adolescents whose parents have gambling problems.

IDENTITY VERSUS ROLE CONFUSION

According to Erik Erikson, a well-known developmental psychologist, adolescence begins at 12 and nears completion at age 18. During the stage known as identity vs. role confusion, adolescents try to establish their identity as young adults. Teenagers often wonder, "What is my role in life?" During this period, young people who have low self-esteem and little confidence may be at an increased risk from negative peer pressure, feeling they must go along with the crowd to prove themselves.

The need to fit in

Many individuals give in to peer pressure because they want to fit in with a particular group. Membership in social groups means sharing the same interests, hobbies, clothes, and ideas of the group as a whole. It is difficult for adolescents to say no when all their friends have already said yes. Some teenagers may fear being disliked or worry about being rejected when they do not go along with their peers' wishes.

Adolescents also may give in to the group out of a sense of curiosity, especially when the pressure to conform relates to something they know very little about. Going along under pressure can be dangerous: it can cloud both their judgment and common sense.

COPING WITH PRESSURE AND STRESS

Stress can cause bodily or mental tension. Adolescence is a vulnerable time, and many young people experience significant negative life events, or stressors, that can cause a great deal of discomfort. Most teens have to learn how to cope with negative emotions, personal relationships, and their involvement in high-risk or addictive behaviors. The impact of life's stressors on the individual depends on duration and intensity. Young people can lessen the effect of these stressful factors by learning coping skills.

Styles of coping

A person's coping skills largely determine how he or she experiences stress. Learning problem-solving skills and focusing on solutions to the many issues adolescents face can lessen the impact of stress on both the individual and others around them.

Task-focused skills: These are strategies that attempt to solve, reconceptualize, or minimize the effects of a stressful situation.

Emotion-focused skills: These include strategies of self-preoccupation, fantasy, or other conscious activities related to the regulation of one's feelings.

Avoidance-focused skills: These are diversion or distraction techniques in which a person engages in alternate tasks, usually activities unrelated to the stressors.

NEGATIVE PEER PRESSURE AND ADOLESCENT GAMBLING

Current research shows that 85 percent of all high school students have gambled in their lifetime, and 73 percent of those 85 percent have gambled in the previous 12 months.

Not only are adolescent gamblers engaging in a risky activity that violates the law, but they also are at an increased risk for conduct problems, binge drinking, suicidal thoughts, multiple sex partners, drug use, and impulse control problems. Current research shows that between 4.4 percent and 7.4 percent of adolescents exhibit signs of pathological gambling behavior, compared to 1 percent to 2 percent of adults. Negative peer pressure, such as someone's making fun of you—for example, for not going along with a risky group activity—can lead to lowered **self-esteem** and depression. In turn, depression in teenagers is a condition that can lead to problem gambling and substance abuse.

VIDEO GAME PLAY AND GAMBLING

Video game playing has long been considered a behavioral addiction in and of itself. Research shows a link between gambling and video game playing, with problem gamblers being more likely to spend excessive amounts of time on game play. The activities are in fact similar, with both providing intermittent rewards and randomness. Studies also show that adolescents who play video games excessively also gamble at least once per week. With 93 percent of households with children reporting that they own at least one gaming console, however, most children report playing video games for excitement and enjoyment.

See also: Adolescents and Gambling; Family Life and Gambling; School and Work Performance and Gambling; Video Gaming

FURTHER READING

Van Cleave, Ryan G. *Unplugged: My Journey into the Dark World of Video Game Addiction.* Deerfield Beach, Fla.: HCI, 2010.

■ PREVENTION AND INTERVENTION

Programs used to help prevent or treat addictive behavior. Prevention involves stopping something before it happens. Intervention is the action of interfering with a behavior in an effort to change an outcome. There are certain things that can help prevent a person from becoming a problem gambler. There are also numerous ways to intervene when a person has already started down the road toward problem gambling. As studies indicate that problem gambling is on the rise, it is important for teens to be aware of what can help protect them.

Because gambling is a popular way to pass time, it is not uncommon to hear about poker parties and gambling tournaments. Although gambling does not involve a mind-altering substance, it is a stimulant and can become highly addictive. Some teens may be at a higher risk than others of becoming addicted to gambling. One precaution is for teens to be aware of certain factors that put them at a higher risk.

RISK FACTORS

According to a 2002 article in the *Journal of Gambling Studies* titled "The Prevention of Gambling Problems in Youth: A Conceptual

Framework," there are many **risk factors** for becoming hooked on gambling. Some of the common risk factors include substance use, being around gambling on a regular basis, hanging out with people who gamble often, and watching gambling on television or over the Internet. One popular form of gambling which is highly publicized is poker. In fact, the World Series of Poker has become such a huge success that many teens look up to the fame and fortune that some poker players possess.

Even if teens find themselves surrounded by such risk factors, however, there are ways for them to protect themselves. For example:

- Avoid using substances.
- Avoid situations where there may be gambling.
- Cut back on or quit hanging out with people who gamble regularly.
- Watch other things on television rather than gambling.

COPING SKILLS

Research reveals that many youth who are involved in problem gambling have unhealthy coping skills. Coping skills are ways that a person handles stressful situations. When a teen is faced with a stressful situation, there are a number of ways he or she might cope with the stressful event. According to the article mentioned in the previous section, coping can be either problem-focused or emotion-oriented. Coping skills also may be active or avoidant.

Problem-focused coping involves directly and actively attempting to resolve the stress or anxiety. Emotion-oriented coping includes things such as daydreaming, constantly thinking about the stressful situation, and emotionally responding to the stress. Research reveals that active coping skills, such as problem-solving and positive thinking result in more positive outcomes. Emotion-oriented coping, on the other hand, tends to lead to more problems.

Some researchers speculate that unhealthy coping skills may lead to problem gambling. Some have found that many people use gambling as a way to mentally escape their stressful situations, which is not a healthy way of coping. Problem-solving a much more effective way of coping, may involve identifying the problem, brainstorming ways to resolve or fix the problem, coming up with a plan, thinking of the possible outcomes of the plan, and then acting on the plan.

EDUCATE YOURSELF

Teens often think irrationally when it comes to gambling. For example, some teens mistakenly believe that gambling is a quick and easy way to make money. The truth is that a person will lose more often than he or she wins. Winning while gambling is a matter of chance—random and unpredictable. Some teens may gamble in order to escape a difficult or boring life situation. The truth is that gambling may lead to more negative consequences than the life being escaped. According to a 2004 article titled "Coping Strategies Employed by Adolescents with Gambling Problems," pathological gambling among adolescents may result in increased crime, problems within family relationships, and poor performance in school.

Q & A

Question: Is there any proven way to guarantee that I won't become a problem gambler?

Answer: Yes, choosing not to gamble at all. Abstaining, or choosing to not gamble, is the only absolute way to ensure that a person will not develop an addiction to gambling.

One common factor that plays a large role in problem gambling is acting on impulse, or in other words, not thinking it all the way through. It is smart to preset limits and to stick with those limits rather than acting impulsively. Some examples of helpful limits may include

- setting a money limit (how much will be spent that day)
- setting a time limit (a specific time to quit gambling or an allotment of time, such as three hours)
- combining the two

If a person goes into a game knowing that he or she will spend "x" amount of money or spend "x" amount of time, that person will be more likely to prevent their gambling from becoming a problem.

Also, be aware of your thoughts. When gambling, a person may experience an intense rush when winning or ahead. However, winning is always momentary and therefore will not last long. It would not be called *gambling* if it were not a gamble, meaning there is NO guarantee that a player will win!

See also: Protective Factors; Risk Taking and Gambling

FURTHER READING
Berman, L., and M. E. Siegal. *BEHIND the 8-BALL: A Recovery Guide for the Families of Gamblers.* New York: iUniverse, 2008.

■ PROTECTIVE FACTORS

Circumstances in life that guard a person from problem situations, in this case, problem gambling. Protective factors help to offset risk factors, which are negative circumstances that may increase a person's engaging in destructive behavior. Although many risk and protective factors are out of your control, there are several that you can control.

AVOID UNNECESSARY RISKS

Inevitably you will be faced with the opportunity to gamble. Gambling is a popular way to pass time. Adolescents may come in contact with poker parties, lotteries, sports betting, horse-race betting, casino games, and many other forms of gambling. Sometimes opportunities to gamble even come from parents and other older individuals whom you look up to. Facing these opportunities and remaining strong in your ability to avoid unnecessary risk is important to avoiding the development of a gambling problem.

Gambling is on the rise throughout the United States. A 2002 article from the *Journal of the Psychology of Addictive Behaviors,* "A Prospective Study of Youth Gambling Behavior," suggests that this rise in legalized gambling plays a role in the increasing number of youth at risk for problem gambling. However, there are a number of things that can help young people prepare to face a gambling situation. Being aware of these ahead of time and working on them before gambling can become a problem will play a role in how you handle gambling now and throughout your life.

DEVELOPMENTAL ASSETS

Building one's personal assets will not only act as a buffer for problem gambling but also help create positive attributes for dealing with life in general. According to the Arizona Office of Problem Gambling, there are 40 protective factors that are considered developmental assets. These assets include

- support
- positive outlook
- realistic boundaries and expectations
- internal control
- high self-esteem
- constructive use of time
- good problem-solving skills

These are factors that a person can incorporate into daily life, attributes that then will serve as a strong foundation for making healthy choices when faced with gambling and other risky situations.

Positive attitudes and behaviors are learned. They are taught in school, on sports teams, in arts programs, in faith-based groups, in family settings, and in many other environments. Everyone should use these learning opportunities to develop a healthy sense of self, a primary asset in avoiding difficult situations such as problem gambling.

Q & A

Question: What is internal control?

Answer: Internal control is also known as having an internal locus of control. This is the psychological concept of the degree to which you feel you have control over your life. People with a lower locus of control believe heavily in chance and luck. Often, this belief results in people feeling that things "happen to" them rather than that they control their surroundings.

A higher locus of control results in better resiliency and ability to handle situations responsibly. Individuals who believe they have more control over their lives possess better adaptability and a stronger sense of self. A high locus of control, or internal control, enables people to choose the best possible path in a situation and actively make choices to improve negative or stressful situations.

GOOD VALUES AND A PERCEIVED POSITIVE ENVIRONMENT

According to the International Center for Youth Gambling Problems and Other High-Risk Behaviors, following are three of the values that will protect and steer teens toward choices that support healthy growth and development and away from potentially addictive behaviors:

- good health
- achievement
- orderly conduct

These values are best supported in an environment that includes, among others, these two protective factors:

- heightened structure
- role models

Living with heightened structure simply means, for example:

- staying on top of daily tasks
- going to bed and waking up at set times
- getting enough rest at night
- eating healthy and regularly
- keeping on top of school assignments

As for role models, find someone who exemplifies your ideas and is living with the values you intend to maintain. A good role model will act as a guide and a defense against problem gambling. Role models do not need to be parents or teachers. A positive role model is anyone who exerts a positive influence—a best friend, a neighbor, a sibling.

Fact Or Fiction?

A role model is someone I have to know personally.

The Facts: A role model can be anyone you look up to. While positive role models can be family members, teachers, friends, or individuals from the community, they also can be famous leaders or politicians, actors, sports stars, or scholars. Role models do not have to be living individuals, simply anyone who has lived in a way you admire and aspire to be like, or "model" yourself after.

THE GOAL IS RESILIENCE

Developing protective factors leads to resilience, which is the ability to cope positively within the context of significant adversity. For example, resilience enables a person to stay strong in the face of peer pressure or overcome a negative home environment, such as living with a parent who is a problem gambler. Adolescents who are able to avoid taking drugs, bullying, and gambling, even when family or friends engage in these negative activities, are resilient.

Seeking help from positive role models can develop resilience. For example, if you do not feel resilient in avoiding peer pressure to gamble, seek help from a teacher or friend who shares your values.

TEENS SPEAK

My Mom Has a Problem

My name is Fiona and I am 15 years old. I live in a one-bedroom apartment with my mom and four brothers and sisters. As much as I'd like my family to have more money and space, this is all I've ever known and it's okay.

My older brother got into drugs real bad, and it tore us apart for a while. My mom gambles too much, and I'm always afraid she will lose our rent money. To me, this is life. I fear for my little brother and sisters, that they too might get into drugs, start gambling, or fail out of school, but I try to be a good role model for them. I think that is what keeps me from falling in.

My school counselor says that I am resilient. I get good grades, and I stay away from the poker parties I get invited to. I guess this is because, even when she's gambling, my mom always stresses the importance of school. My younger siblings and I have a pretty structured schedule, and we keep to it every school day—dinner at 6:00, then homework, and lights out at 9:30. I think this combination of achieving good reports at school and taking responsibility at home keeps me resilient. Other kids in similar situations should know that no matter how bad life sometimes seems, if you stick to your values and stay away from drugs, alcohol, and gambling, you'll come out on the other side unscathed.

See also: Adolescents and Gambling; Family Life and Gambling; Help for Gamblers; Prevention and Intervention; Risk Taking and Gambling.

FURTHER READING
Hugel, Bob. *I Did It Without Thinking: True Stories About Impulsive Decisions That Changed Lives.* New York: Children's Press, 2008.
Sojourner, Mary. *She Bets Her Life: A True Story of Gambling Addiction.* Berkeley, Calif.: Seal Press, 2010.

■ PUBLIC HEALTH ISSUES AND GAMBLING

Topics that affect the well-being of society at large with a concentration on prevention, harm reduction, creating awareness, and early interventions. Due to the rising percentage of problem gamblers, gambling is very much a public health issue. It affects every aspect of society, relationships, economics, and personal health.

PREVENTION AND HARM REDUCTION

Public health officials and agencies seek to prevent or reduce problem behavior with screenings for early detection, as well as by creating awareness of certain issues. Unfortunately, there is currently a lack of prevention or education programs targeted toward problem gambling awareness.

Screenings are short questionnaires that assess and identify a problem behavior. In order to identify people who might need help, screenings should be conducted at hospitals, clinics, mental health centers, or schools prior to recommending more extensive evaluation and potential treatment by clinical professionals. Often, a gambling addiction mimics drug addiction; however, if a gambling screening is not completed the addiction goes untreated. There are several types of screening tools used to identify problem gamblers. Those tools used most often are: the *DSM-IV* Pathological Gambling Diagnostic Form; the South Oaks Gambling Screen (SOGS); The NORC *DSM-IV* Screen for Gambling Problems; the Gamblers Anonymous 20 questions; and the Lie/Bet assessment.

SCREENING TOOLS

The *Diagnostic and Statistical Manual of Mental Disorders-IV (DSM-IV)*, Pathological Gambling Diagnostic Form, is based on the *DSM* criteria for pathological gamblers. The form asks questions that directly correlate to the 10 symptoms covered in the *DSM-IV*. This assessment is usually used in conjunction with another assessment form to confirm the diagnosis.

The South Oaks Gambling Screen is based on the problem gambling criteria found in the *Diagnostic and Statistical Manual of Mental Disorders-III-R*. The South Oaks Gambling Screen is an assessment that consists of 20 questions. The assessment was designed to identify individuals with a lifetime incidence of problem gambling. Experts consider the South Oaks Gambling Screen to be one of the best and most reliable screening tools.

The NORC *DSM-IV* Screen for Gambling Problems (NORC) is a screening assessment created by the National Opinion Research Center. This tool consists of 17 questions and is based on the *DSM-IV* criteria for pathological gambling. The purpose of this assessment is to identify problem gamblers in the general population. The NORC lists five levels of problem gambler:

- Type A: The individual is not a gambler.
- Type B: The individual is a low-risk gambler, never betting more than $100 in a year.
- Type C: The individual meets one or two of the *DSM-IV* criteria for pathological gambling.
- Type D: The individual meets three or four of the *DSM-IV* criteria for pathological gambling.
- Type E: The individual meets five or more of the *DSM-IV* criteria for pathological gambling.

The Gamblers Anonymous 20 questions are typically issued to an individual when he or she attends Gamblers Anonymous group sessions. On this assessment, answering *yes* to at least seven questions indicates a gambling problem.

PERSONAL HEALTH PROBLEMS

Gambling negatively affects health. Problems include depression, anxiety, insomnia, intestinal disorders, and migraines. These physical symptoms are the result of stress and possibly of withdrawal. The cessation of gambling can cause physical withdrawal symptoms similar to those felt when stopping the use of drugs like crack or cocaine. These symptoms include sleeplessness, headaches, weakness, heart palpitations, muscle aches, dizziness, and shortness of breath. Because the symptoms of problem gambling are not always obvious, the signs of addiction often go unnoticed by the individual, family, or friends before the problem has advanced into a chronic addiction.

Interventions for gambling addiction are similar to those in other addiction recovery programs. Problem gamblers may receive inpatient and/or outpatient rehabilitation as well as individual and group counseling. Problem gamblers also can seek help by utilizing twelve-step programs. Gamblers Anonymous is such a program, similar to Alcoholics Anonymous but designed for gamblers by gamblers.

FAMILY AND SOCIAL PROBLEMS

Gambling affects a person's family and social life as negatively as it affects one's health. Problem gamblers lie about how much they spend and how they spend their time. Gambling almost never begins as tragically as it ends. Gamblers "chase" their losses, which means for every bet they lose, they bet more and more to make up for the money lost. Because gambling is so risky, an individual may never make up the loss, and with each bet placed, he or she falls more and more into debt. This may result in a person's blowing through entire savings, taking out another mortgage, or using one's tuition savings for a child's college education.

Often friends and family do not notice this behavior until it is too late. One of the major causes of divorce is disagreement over money. Problem gamblers need to increase their wager, or bet, to feel the same rush each time they gamble, which results in increasing amounts of debt. Gambling debt also may result in legal problems. Gamblers may feel the need to steal from family, friends, or employers. Although a gambler usually takes money with the intention of repaying it, the need to gamble more for the rush or chasing the loss often results in the gambler's inability to repay stolen funds.

The physical changes in a gambler also affect social and family life. Depression, for example, may make it hard for the individual to spend time with family and friends. Common signs of depression include problems sleeping, a loss of appetite or overeating, loss of enjoyment in activities that the gambler previously enjoyed, and difficulty concentrating.

PEOPLE WHO ARE AT RISK

Public health approaches also include focusing on populations at risk for developing problems. Those groups most at risk for developing problem gambling are: adolescents, the elderly, substance-dependent individuals, and individuals from a low social and economic background.

Teens at risk

Adolescents are at risk for developing problem gambling because of the experimental and novelty-seeking aspects that are normal in their developmental level. Research indicates that while only 1 to 2 percent of the adult population are problem gamblers, 4 to 8 percent of the adolescent population are problem gamblers. Problem gambling in adolescents often goes unnoticed because of the lack of physical symptoms. Teen gamblers have a higher risk of depression, substance abuse, suicide, and anxiety and more problems with health in general.

Seniors and the elderly

People over 70 are at risk for developing problem gambling because they are often socially isolated. Trips to a casino can act as a way to socialize or be around other people. Gambling can be an escape from the loneliness and isolation that often occurs when children move out of the home or a spouse dies.

Socio-economic status

Although households in a higher social or income bracket spend more per year than do those of lower socioeconomic status, research has shown that people with less money or social standing spend proportionately more on gambling.

Substance abusers

Individuals who abuse drugs, alcohol, or tobacco are also at risk for developing problems with gambling. Drugs and alcohol lower inhibitions and may cause individuals to bet more than they intended. This is why many casinos offer free alcoholic drinks to people who gamble in their establishments. Substance abuse can be either a leading factor for beginning to gamble or a result of gambling.

CONCLUSIONS

Gambling has many negative effects on public health. It tears families apart, ruins social relationships, and can result in legal problems. Prevention and harm reduction can lower the risk and incidence of problem gambling. Also, screenings and early interventions with treatment can reduce the development of problem gambling and assist people in getting help.

See also: Adolescents and Gambling; Prevention and Intervention; Protective Factors

FURTHER READING
Messerlian, C., and R. Derevensky. "Youth Gambling Problems: A Public Health Perspective." *Health Promotion International* (2005).

■ RISK TAKING AND GAMBLING

A risk is any action for which there is some possibility of failure as well as some opportunity for success. Risk taking means making a decision to participate in a behavior that may have either a positive or a negative outcome. For example, if a person decides to gamble, he or she is choosing risk over a certain outcome.

Every day, people make decisions that can be positive and successful or negative and unsuccessful. Risk and risk taking are universal experiences that experts believe are essential for healthy growth and development. In fact, risk taking appears to fulfill a lot of important psychosocial needs, as it

- builds self-confidence
- enhances self-esteem

- promotes autonomy
- builds self-identity
- helps a person to gain peer acceptance and respect

Risk is inescapable. It is everywhere—driving in traffic, breathing city air, expressing one's views. People take risks every day—when they must make decisions about career choices, whether or not to marry, where to live. Attempting to avoid one kind of risk may back us into another. Cutting back on nuclear power reduces the risk of radioactive accidents, but burning more fossil fuel increases acid rain and global warming.

TYPES OF RISKS

Risks may be physical, psychological, social, emotional, or financial in nature. Risk taking may be constructive (positive) or destructive (negative), depending on the outcome of the risk-taking behavior and how it affects one's health. Adolescents and adults pursue risks and risk taking as a normal part of living.

Motivation for risk taking

Adolescents engage in risky behavior as the result of a complex interplay of factors, including

- body chemistry
- brain development
- cognitive growth
- culture
- nutrition

Adolescents and adults take risks for adventure, to escape boredom, or to feel excitement, as well as to have the opportunity to experience success and novelty. Those who gamble in casinos, play the state lottery, go to horror movies, choose to ride wild roller coasters at amusement parks, consume alcohol and other drugs, bungee jump, invest in the stock market, and have promiscuous sex have one thing in common. They are taking risks, pursuing thrills (sensation seeking), and experiencing physical and neurobiological arousal. One feels a "chemical brain rush" when doing something that is unpredictable but also intense. The motivation for risk taking is driven by biological, psychological, and social factors.

Motivation for youth gambling

Gambling is an example of risky behavior. Young people participate in gambling for many different reasons. While gambling can be fun and exciting, it also can be scary and stressful when a person loses money as well as control of his or her behavior. Teenagers may participate in gambling in order to cope with other life issues, as well as to seek activities that appear to provide temporary excitement, pleasure, and an escape from boredom and personal problems.

THE RISK OF ADDICTION

Gambling can be addictive due to its influence on brain chemicals such as serotonin and dopamine, which provide a sense of pleasure and a temporary sense of well-being. Although they are underage, youth have abundant opportunities to engage in gambling through the Internet, state and national lotteries, gambling machines, sports betting, playing card games like poker, and video gaming.

As with any other compulsive disorders, problem or compulsive gamblers experience an escalation in risk-taking behavior. The gambler gets hooked on the thrill that he or she feels after winning, only to have it followed by a slow decline into the despair of losing. At this point, the gambler can no longer rationalize his behavior. However, instead of taking a step back and looking at the problem logically, the person hopes to repeat the original "rush" of feelings and cannot stop the destructive behavior. He or she tricks himself or herself into thinking that just hitting that one big jackpot could make everything right again. This sounds good and temporarily reduces the anxiety about losses and debts. Eventually, however, the person develops a harmful dependency on the original feelings. Until something happens that creates panic, the problem escalates.

Caught in this dynamic, the compulsive gambler experiences greater and greater negative consequences: legal problems, damaged or severed relationships, abuse of alcohol or drugs, suicidal thoughts or attempts. Typically, a final crisis leads to the admission of defeat. Then, and only then, does the compulsive gambler tend to seek help.

Problem gambling also has an impact on public and personal health. Problem gambling is associated with a number of other unhealthy adolescent risky behaviors such as involvement in unprotected sex, drugs, alcohol, tobacco, emotional problems, and delinquency.

Risky Problem Behaviors and Adolescent Health

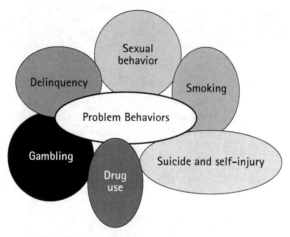

Research shows that adolescent problem gambling typically co-occurs with other risky behaviors and that these problem behaviors, particularly in combination, negatively impact emotional health and stability.

HEALTHY RISK PROMOTION

Both young people and adults should be encouraged to participate in adventurous, sensation-seeking, exhilarating experiences that fulfill one's needs and that are healthy and legal. These activities are constructive risk taking.

Healthy Risks

According to psychologist Joseph Ilardo, risk taking for personal growth may include:

1. Self-improvement Risks

   These are any actions taken to improve or develop oneself as a person.

   Examples include returning to school as an adult; mastering a skill (learning an instrument or a sport, creating art); trying out for a part in a play or orchestra; entering therapy; attending a Gamblers Anonymous meeting or other self-help group; volunteering for a challenging assignment on the job or in the community; trying out for a competitive scholarship or award.

2. Commitment Risks

   These are any actions that involve putting oneself on the line on behalf of a higher cause or value.

   Examples include contributing to a cause, charity, or political campaign; volunteering to work for a cause, charity, candidate; joining a movement or organization; marrying or establishing a monogamous relationship; having or adopting a baby; lobbying for change, such as writing to one's senator or leading a protest movement.

3. Self-disclosure Risks

   These are any actions that result in others knowing your wants, likes, feelings, preferences, goals.

   Examples include assertive behavior, including expressing one's feelings when attracted to someone; confronting someone with whom you are upset; making one's wants known without apologizing; openly supporting an unpopular cause; confessing some flaw, character trait, or quality others might not know about; questioning or challenging a standing policy or an authority;

DID YOU KNOW?

Constructive Risk Taking

Unhealthy Risks

Youth Risk Taking

Healthy Risk Promotion

Healthy Risks

The challenge of healthy risk promotion is to channel youth risk taking into positive, health-enhancing experiences and to provide realistic alternative options to destructive behavior.

starting a conversation with a stranger; asking someone out on a date.

Finding a balance

Risk taking is necessary for healthy functioning. Health, for most people, is a matter of balancing risks, rather than taking none at all! Effective interventions entail encouraging those risks that are developmentally appropriate and providing opportunities for young people to acquire healthy skills acquisition and develop social bonding to others who are exhibiting pro-social (rather than antisocial) behaviors.

Healthy risk taking is a positive tool in an adolescent's life for discovering, developing, and consolidating his or her identity. Adolescent risk taking becomes negative only when the risks are dangerous, for example, when engaging in behavior that could lead to problem gambling. Healthy risks—often understood as "challenges"—can turn unhealthy risks in a more positive direction, or prevent them from ever taking place.

ASSESSING RISKS

Adolescents need both support and tools to be able to assess risks and move from unhealthy risk taking to healthy risk taking. In order to undertake healthy alternatives to dangerous risk taking, adolescents need the active help and support of the adults in their lives, including parents and school health professionals. It is important to remember that learning how to assess risks is a process that we work on throughout our lives.

Healthy risks provide opportunities for enjoyment, pleasure, and ways to cope with life's challenges. Successful engagement in activities such as those in the table of "Healthy Alternatives" helps one feel good, improves self-esteem, and affords chances to make friends and interact in positive social networks.

See also: Adolescents and Gambling; Peer Pressure and Gambling; Protective Factors

FURTHER READING

Ilardo, J. *Risk-Taking for Personal Growth*. Oakland, Calif.: New Harbinger Publications, Inc., 1992.

Jordan-Wyatt, T., and Fred Peterson. "Risky Business: Exploring Adolescent Risk-Taking Behavior." *Journal of School Health* (August 2005).

Healthy Alternatives to Dangerous Behavior

UNHEALTHY RISK BEHAVIORS	HEALTHY RISK BEHAVIORS
Dangerous dieting, eating disorders	Physical activities such as sports teams, horseback riding, skating, walking, jogging, or working out
Using drugs, alcohol, steroids	*Under the supervision of a trained expert,* engaging in outlets for extreme physical and emotional thrills such as whitewater rafting, rock climbing, camping; creative activities such as joining a band or the production of a play
Running away, staying out all night, living on the streets	Learning or practicing a creative art form such as photography, pottery, video, dance, creative writing
Unprotected sexual activity	Learning to talk about sex and relationships; working on open communication with partners and parents
Gang violence, weapons, bullying, scapegoating	Seeking out new friends, volunteering in the community, participating in a student exchange program, transferring to a new school if necessary
Shoplifting, stealing	Getting a part-time job such as babysitting, camp or after-school counselor, retail clerk in clothing or music store, tutoring
Suicide, self-injury	Finding an enjoyable and pleasurable hobby such as taking care of pets, raising rabbits or other animals, working on a farm
Gambling	Becoming involved in activities that fulfill the need for thrill- or sensation-seeking and that are healthy and legal

Source: Adapted July 2010 from Lynn Ponton, *The Romance of Risk—Why Teenagers Do the Things They Do.* New York: Basic Books, 1997.

According to psychiatrist Lynn E. Ponton, all of the healthy risks in the right-hand column are suggestions of healthy alternatives to the unhealthy behaviors in the left-hand column.

■ SCHOOL AND WORK PERFORMANCE AND GAMBLING

The relationship between academic and job performance and gaming behavior, in which a person chooses risk over a certain outcome. Gambling can infiltrate every aspect of a person's life. It starts as entertainment and often leads to a life of lies and cover-ups.

Gambling affects social relationships negatively. The addiction can cause individuals to create rifts in family relationships as well as relationships with friends. The detrimental effects on relationships also damage work and school life. Not only do pathological gamblers erode relationships with schoolmates and peers at work, but they also tend to break the law.

ADOLESCENTS AND THE LAW

For adolescents, gambling is illegal and attendance at school is a law. If an individual does not attend school, he or she is truant and faces penalties from both school and law enforcement. Also, gambling on school property may lead to stiff punishment by one's institution.

The work environment is affected differently. If an individual does not show up to work, he or she faces corrective action such as suspension or termination. Naturally, job loss can have detrimental effects on an individual and the individual's family. Furthermore, studies have shown that gambling often leads to stealing from one's place of employment, an offense that carries a likely penalty of imprisonment.

PATHOLOGICAL GAMBLING AND SCHOOL PERFORMANCE

Young people with gambling problems tend to have numerous arguments with family members. These conflicts may be due to money problems, lying, poor work performance, low grades, stealing, and irresponsibility in general. Problem gamblers tend to lie to cover up their losses and to obtain money for further gambling. Once the family realizes the constant lies, they tend to argue with the gambler, which in turn affects the individual's school performance. In addition to poor attendance, the stress of having problems at home often interferes with the person's ability to concentrate on academic tasks and assignments. The more stress a problem gambler experiences, the more he is likely to gamble, increasing the problems at home. In other words, this addictive behavior creates a vicious cycle.

Q & A

Question: If I am expelled from school for gambling, does that mean I cannot go to another school?

Answer: Expulsion means that a person cannot attend the school from which he or she was removed. Sometimes, that student also cannot attend any other school in the same district without a school board hearing. If you are expelled from a private school, you should be able to attend another private school. However, an expulsion remains on your school record and may impede your ability to get into college.

Because their priority is to gamble, gamblers tend to have poor grades and low attendance. This unhealthy behavior affects the student's ability to complete school tasks and participate in extra-curricular activities, all of which jeopardizes the completion of a high school or college degree. Therefore, graduation rates among gamblers are significantly low.

Pathological gamblers tend to engage in gambling with their peers during school hours. This can cause serious problems, such as:

- Gambling inside of a school is against school policy. If students gamble, they face penalties such as detention, suspension, or expulsion.
- Fights and arguments are common. This is because of money problems or bad relationships with peers. In turn, fights can lead to suspension or expulsion.
- The pathological gambler may engage in other illegal activities at school in order to obtain money for gambling.
- Expulsion tends to result in failure to graduate.

PATHOLOGICAL GAMBLING AND WORK PERFORMANCE

Job performance is highly affected by an employee's problem gambling. This behavior often results in citations, suspension, or loss of work. Not only will gamblers miss work often, but also the loss of money from less employment leads the individual to gamble more and falsely believe that he or she will make up that loss.

Gamblers also tend to steal in the workplace, usually to be able to afford their gambling or to pay off their debts. Surprisingly, many individuals do not consider taking money from their workplace to be stealing. They wrongly imagine that they will take money to gamble, double the amount borrowed, and then return the money. This risky negative and illegal behavior leads to more debt, often job loss, and even imprisonment.

Personal relationships at work are also affected by pathological gambling behaviors. For example, if one owes money to several coworkers, the situation can result in isolation—and eventually termination.

Productivity over treatment

Employers are more concerned with the productivity of their employees than with helping them overcome their addictions. Therefore, employers usually dismiss any employee who cannot keep up with the work. It is much more cost effective for an employer to dismiss employees than it is to pay for their treatment, provide extra days off, or any other considerations. It is for this reason that pathological gamblers tend to lose their jobs. Also, although most companies that offer insurance to their employees offer mental health coverage, which includes treatment for addiction, pathological gambling is not often considered an addiction or a diagnosis covered by insurance companies. Therefore, companies tend to look at pathological gambling as the employee's problem alone.

CONCLUSION

Clearly, pathological gamblers typically do not perform to their full potential. This may be explained as gamblers focus their attention on gambling and not on other tasks. They become highly preoccupied with the next gambling event and not on work or school.

Pathological gambling affects all aspects of the gambler's life and slowly takes away necessary support systems. More research is needed for this problem, and employers and school personnel should consider that because addictions negatively affect most people directly or indirectly, they should address the problem. Finally, more treatment programs need to be established in order to effectively help the pathological gambler.

See also: Addiction and Gambling; Binge Gambling; Family Life and Gambling; Law and Gambling, The; Youth at Special Risk

FURTHER READING
Griffiths, Mark. *Adolescent Gambling.* Adolescence and Society Series. New York: Routledge, 1995.
Silverman Saunders, Carol. *Straight Talk About Teenage Gambling.* New York: Facts On File, 1999.

SOCIAL GAMBLING

Generally viewed as gaming for entertainment only. Gambling and games of chance have been popular activities in most societies and cultures throughout history. However, despite gambling's continuous popularity among individuals, societies themselves have taken a variety of views of this risk-taking activity. For example, in the United States, gambling has transitioned from prohibition to widespread proliferation. It has evolved from being associated with sin, criminal behavior, and corruption to its current position as a form of socially acceptable entertainment.

MORE PEOPLE GAMBLE TODAY

Once considered an undesirable activity by many Americans, gambling is being increasingly embraced as socially acceptable. For example, in 1975, the proportion of adults who reported that they "never gambled" was one in three, or approximately 33 percent of the adult population. Today, the number of adults who have reported that they "never gambled" has decreased to one in seven, or approximately 15 percent of the adult population.

In fact, over the past 20 years, gambling has become a major global industry. Statistics indicate that approximately 85 percent of all American adults have gambled at least once in their lives, and 65–80 percent reported having gambled in the past year. These numbers are quite similar to the research results cited in Canada, Australia, and New Zealand.

Prior to 1989, Nevada and Atlantic City were the only two U.S. jurisdictions with legalized casino gambling. Since then, legalized casino-style gaming has grown throughout the country: on American Indian reservations, in limited-stakes casinos in South Dakota and Colorado, and on riverboats in Iowa, Illinois, Mississippi, and Louisiana. In fact, all but two U.S. states—Hawaii and Utah—feature some form of legalized gambling.

THE GROWTH OF THE GAMBLING INDUSTRY

Many factors have contributed to the gaming industry's unprecedented growth. Increases in people's disposable income and leisure time contribute to gambling's popularity. Also, the expansion of state-run lotteries has been an influential factor. Both permitted and promoted by many jurisdictions, lotteries have become a major source of income for state and local governments. As is seen with federal and local laws that permit and even encourage gambling, new gaming venues, new forms of gambling (for example, new technologies in the form of interactive lotteries, Internet gambling, telephone wagering), and the proliferation of current forms of gambling (such as casinos or riverboats) will continue to be supported.

Additionally, the gaming industry itself has done its best to nurture its own growth by highlighting the positive economic and social effects of gambling. For example, gambling venues create jobs, and tax revenues derived from gambling support government services.

Gambling is promoted almost everywhere as fun, glamorous, and exciting. Advertising and marketing campaigns depict gambling as an activity that tests daring, skill, courage, intelligence, and luck. The gaming industry has been so successful in their marketing of gambling that today gaming represents the largest segment of the overall American entertainment industry. Consumers spend more on legal gambling in the United States than they do on all other forms of entertainment, more than on music, movies, and theater combined.

THE SOCIAL APPEAL

Gambling appeals to people's inherent risk-taking nature as well as their social nature. In a 1985 publication, *When Luck Runs Out*, Robert Custer and Harry Milt capture the social appeal of gambling:

In addition to the chance of winning, gambling also offers for many the opportunity to socialize. For these people, the bingo game in the basement of a church or a card game at the country club once or twice a week is a major social activity. The crowd at the OTB (Off-Track Betting) office shares a feeling of fraternity. . . . The local Friday-night poker game has, for millions of Americans, become a traditional social function. . . . [E]ven the thousands of transients who mill about the gambling casinos of Las Vegas and other venues nightly enjoy a sense of camaraderie and belonging, a feeling of being comfortable and safe.

WHY PEOPLE GAMBLE

According to the results of a Harvard Medical School survey, in order of popularity, the following list represents the primary reasons that people gamble:

- to win money
- for entertainment
- for excitement
- for curiosity
- to socialize
- for a worthy cause
- as a distraction
- as a hobby

TYPES OF GAMBLERS

Gambling behavior falls along a continuum. On one end of the continuum lies social gambling, generally viewed as harmless. On the other end of the continuum lies pathological gambling, which carries with it numerous significant negative consequences. According to author Robert Custer, the following are the six types of gamblers:

Casual social gambler

As the label indicates, this type of gambler is one who does not experience problems from gambling. Gambling may be a regular activity, such as periodic, recreational trips to a casino or purchasing a weekly lottery ticket. The casual social gambler would not lose more than intended nor find it difficult to stop gambling. Social gamblers are adults who maintain control over the time, money, and energy that they expend on gambling. They consider the cost of gambling to be payment for entertainment.

Heavy social gambler

While this gambler may rarely lose more money than intended, he or she spends a large amount of time gambling or on gambling-related activities. For example, someone involved with sports betting might spend hours reviewing point spreads, injury reports, scouting reports, and trades in order to make so-called educated bets. The gambling and associated behavior of this type of gambler can impact vocational function and family relationships because of the extensive amount of time spent preparing for gambling and following the bets, namely watching the games.

Professional gambler

This type of gambler is relatively rare and is not usually considered one who has a gambling problem. They control the amount of time spent gambling and the amount of money wagered.

Antisocial gambler

Also rare, this is an individual who is involved in cheating—marking cards, rigging slot machines, and so on—in order to win.

Relief-and-escape gambler

Also characterized as a problem gambler, this individual gambles in order to escape life's problems or situations. Problem gamblers may be lonely, anxious, or depressed. As a result, they may gamble as a way to numb themselves against uncomfortable feelings. This behavior is similar to the way that some people abuse alcohol or other drugs in order to temporarily dull unpleasant emotions.

Compulsive/pathological gambler

These individuals are preoccupied with both gambling and securing money in order to gamble. They cannot control the amount of time or money spent on gambling. To the compulsive or pathological gambler, gambling becomes the most important or most central aspect of that individual's life. The compulsive/pathological gambler may engage in illegal activities in order to acquire the money to gamble.

UNDERAGE GAMBLING

While gambling was once perceived as an activity primarily relegated to adults, it has become a popular form of entertainment for teens. However, adolescent gambling violates the law. Most state and other statutes prohibit children and adolescents from participating in any form of gambling, including legalized gambling. Therefore, when youth do find ways to gamble, it is always a problem, because underage gambling is, by definition, illegal.

Most adolescents are best described as social gamblers. However, from 4 to 8 percent of adolescents have developed a very serious gambling problem. Additionally, statistics indicate that another 10–15 percent are at risk for developing a gambling problem. Although most people can gamble without incurring negative consequences, adolescent social gamblers appear to be more vulnerable to developing a gambling problem than do adult social gamblers.

Increased risk for teens

From a developmental perspective, there are a number of variables associated with an adolescent's increased susceptibility for developing a gambling disorder. Adolescence represents a time of significant physiological, cognitive, and emotional changes; feelings of insecurity; increases in risk-taking behaviors; and a drive for greater independence and autonomy. The inherent tendency for risk taking, a perceived sense of invulnerability, and a limited awareness of gambling-related problems or the negative consequences associated with gambling all combine to increase an adolescent's risk for developing a gambling problem. In fact, a National Research Council report indicates that the prevalence of pathological gamblers among adolescents in the United States could be as much as three times higher than that of adults. Furthermore, research shows that more than 90 percent of those people identified as problem and/or pathological gamblers began gambling in their mid-teens.

Generally speaking, most adolescents who engage in some gambling activities, although breaking the law, will not experience adverse consequences as a result. However, those adolescents who become preoccupied with gambling may develop problem or pathological gambling disorders that may lead to long-lasting negative consequences in their academic standing, interpersonal relationships, psychological development, and general mental and physical health, as well as have consequences arising from engaging in criminal behavior. Additionally, some researchers suggest that disordered gambling not only may be problematic in and of itself, but it also may serve as a gateway to alcohol and substance abuse, depression, anxiety, and other significant mental health disorders.

See also: Addiction and Gambling; Adolescents and Gambling; Gambling, History of; Law and Gambling, The; Peer Pressure and Gambling; Protective Factors; Risk Taking and Gambling

FURTHER READING

Derevensky, Jeffrey, and Rina Gupta. *Gambling Problems in Youth: Theoretical and Applied Perspectives.* New York: Kluwer Academic Publishers, 2004.

Essau, Cecilia A. *Adolescent Addiction: Epidemiology, Assessment, and Treatment.* London: Elsevier, 2008.

Lezine, DeQuincy. *Eight Stories Up: An Adolescent Chooses Hope over Suicide.* Oxford: Oxford University Press, 2008.

■ SPORTS GAMBLING

According to the national self-help organization Gamblers Anonymous, gambling occurs any time there is betting or wagering, for self or others, whether with money or not, no matter how slight or insignificant, where the outcome is uncertain or depends on chance or "skill." Every time you bet money on something, even if it is only a few dollars wagering that your school is going to win the championship game, you are gambling, that is, choosing a risk over a certain outcome.

When most people think about sports and gambling, they probably envision people sitting at a casino slot machine or a group of guys sitting around playing poker. However, there are many other types of sports gambling: horse-racing, dog-racing, collegiate and professional sports, to name a few. In fact, in 1999, following the last official study, the National Gambling Impact Study Commission reported that somewhere between $80 billion and $380 billion is bet illegally on sports in the United States each year.

Q & A

Question: Which of the following is considered a form of sports gambling?

- **buying a raffle ticket at school**
- **creating a pool for the NCAA playoffs**
- **wagering on a high school's championship game**

Answer: All of the above. These are all forms of sports gambling. Remember, gambling occurs any time money is risked to try to win more money.

ATHLETES AND GAMBLING

Athletes, even good athletes, have been known to gamble illegally, where they "throw" a game to ensure a loss. In 2006, for example, three basketball and three football players from the University of Toledo were charged with conspiracy to commit sports bribery. The players accepted between $500 and $1,000 from two bookies for **shaving points** during their games. The wagers totaled $407,500, a serious offense. In baseball, once–star player Pete Rose not only served time in prison for illegal gambling, but he also admitted to and sought treatment for his gambling addiction to betting on baseball in the 1980s.

Art Schlichter, a famous and first-rate quarterback who played for the Ohio State Buckeyes from 1978 to 1981, got snared in the dangerous web of sports betting and succumbed to gambling addiction. In his obsession with gambling, he channeled through the three phases of problem gambling:

1. **Winning or adventurous phase: the search for action or escape** Fun, exciting, entertaining, and rewarding with occasional big wins; unreasonable optimism; fantasies about the big win

2. **Losing phase: the chase** Consistent losses and increased preoccupation with gambling, selling personal possessions; borrowing to bet; personality changes; gambling to recoup losses (called "chasing the bet"); missing work

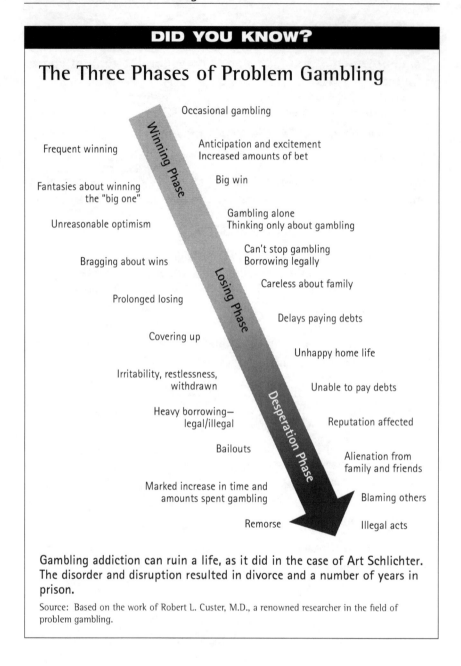

DID YOU KNOW?

The Three Phases of Problem Gambling

Occasional gambling

Frequent winning

Winning Phase

Anticipation and excitement
Increased amounts of bet

Big win

Fantasies about winning
the "big one"

Unreasonable optimism

Gambling alone
Thinking only about gambling

Can't stop gambling
Borrowing legally

Bragging about wins

Losing Phase

Careless about family

Prolonged losing

Delays paying debts

Covering up

Unhappy home life

Irritability, restlessness,
withdrawn

Unable to pay debts

Heavy borrowing—
legal/illegal

Desperation Phase

Reputation affected

Bailouts

Alienation from
family and friends

Marked increase in time and
amounts spent gambling

Blaming others

Remorse

Illegal acts

Gambling addiction can ruin a life, as it did in the case of Art Schlichter. The disorder and disruption resulted in divorce and a number of years in prison.

Source: Based on the work of Robert L. Custer, M.D., a renowned researcher in the field of problem gambling.

3. Desperation phase: panic and the end of the line
   Stealing or other criminal activity to cover bets

People and things to avoid

Following are terms you may know but that are usually associated with illegal sports betting:

- bookie–This person accepts cash bets on a particular outcome. If that outcome is correct, then the bookie gives a payout to the gambler.

- point shaving–This occurs when money is promised to an athlete who ensures his or her team will either lose or not cover the point spread.

- point spread–This type of betting occurs when the gambler is not just interested in whether or not a team will win or lose but instead by how many points that team will win or lose.

Consequences

If a person gets caught illegally placing bets on sports or is involved in a point-shaving scandal, the charges can be very serious. They may include but are not limited to **money laundering,** conspiracy, promoting gambling, and fraud. That person also could face up to 25 years in prison.

HOW SPORTS GAMBLING AFFECTS TEENS

When a child or teen begins gambling, it may seem innocent. However, this behavior can spiral out of control very quickly. The first few times a person wins, it is very exciting. Typically, however, bets get bigger and eventually people bet more money than they have. Like getting a taste of their favorite candy, they cannot get enough.

Even young gamblers start borrowing money from family and friends. When they cannot borrow any more money, they begin to do whatever they can to get money to pay back debts and then bet more money. This is called "chasing the debt." For example, a person bets $5 and loses. Then, that person bets $10, thinking, "I can win and get back my initial $5 bet." This is usually *not* the case. Instead, this is an unhealthy risky behavior with a negative outcome.

Risk Factors

According to psychologist Jon E. Grant, in a 2004 report, adolescent gamblers tend to

- be male
- come from a non-white racial group and a non-traditional household
- have one or more parents who gamble
- have used marijuana in the past year

Fact Or Fiction?

If you're good at strategy games, you will probably be good at figuring out the spread of a game.

The Facts: Unlike a strategy game, one *cannot* actually predict the outcome of a sporting event.

HOW PREVALENT IS IT?

The available research offers only a small window into a wide world of sports gambling. Betting is usually done in a secretive way; therefore, unless a person gets caught in the act, it is difficult to track the occurrences. For example:

- According to a 2008 report, 2.1 percent of NCAA college basketball players claimed to have been asked by gamblers to "fix," or throw, games.
- In 1999, 0.4 percent of NCAA basketball players claimed to have accepted money for performing poorly in a game.

Estimates indicate that collegiate gambling is increasingly prevalent today. In fact, according to Dan Romer, director of the Annenberg Adolescent Risk Communication Institute at the University of Pennsylvania, in 2008, 26.4 percent of young men reported betting on sports on a monthly basis, up from 20.7 percent in 2007.

TREATMENT INTERVENTIONS

If someone has a gambling problem, here are some things that can help:

- group counseling. Sitting down with a group of people one's own age can help a person recognize and avoid triggers that set off the gambling behavior. This is

DID YOU KNOW?

Student Athlete Gambling Activities While Attending College

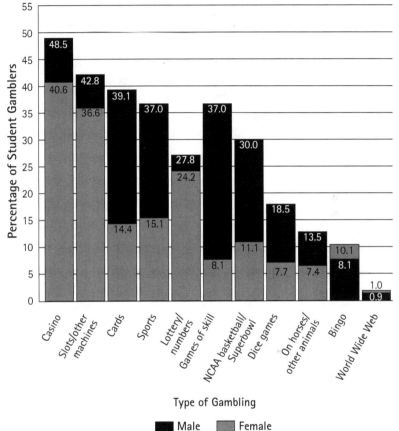

Type of Gambling

■ Male ▨ Female

As seen in the chart, 37 percent of 758 male and female students in a University of Michigan study reported being involved with sports gambling. Although the study only surveyed a relatively small number of students, it puts into perspective how widespread it is that young adults participate in sports gambling.

Source: Adapted from data by Cross, Michael E., and Ann G. Vollano. "The Extent and Nature of Gambling Among College Student Athletes." University of Michigan Department of Athletics, 1999.

also a great way to build a support network and make new friends. Gamblers Anonymous and Gam-anon are two twelve-step groups that help gamblers and their families. These groups can be found in most cities and have proven helpful for many individuals, especially when paired with individual counseling.

- individual counseling. A professional counselor or therapist can set up treatment plans that cater to a person's specific needs and allow the gambler to explore ways to change impulsive behaviors. Seeking help is the first step toward a gambling-free life.

See also: Addiction and Gambling; Gambling, History of; Risk Taking and Gambling

FURTHER READING

Barthelme, Fredrick, and Steven Barthelme. *Double Down: Reflections on Gambling and Loss.* New York: Mariner Books, 2001.

Marotta, Jeffery J. *The Downside: Problem and Pathological Gambling.* Reno: University of Nevada/Reno Bureau of Business, 2002.

Schlichter, Arthur, and J. Snook. *Busted: The Rise and Fall of Art Schlichter.* Wilmington, Ohio: Orange Frazer Press, 2009.

■ SUICIDE AND GAMBLING

The relationship between taking one's own life and gambling. Suicide has been characterized as a human response to extreme physical and/ or prolonged psychological pain. Chronic physical illnesses, terminal diagnoses, prolonged periods of depression and hopelessness, substance abuse, and gambling disorders all have been linked to suicide. Most individuals who experience these challenges do not engage in acts of violence against themselves, or suicide; however, severe problems—such as being a problem or pathological gambler—make some individuals more vulnerable to either contemplating suicide or actually attempting suicide.

SUICIDE RATES AND TENDENCIES

Although the overall rate of suicide among teens has been on the decline since 1992, it is estimated that an adolescent or young adult commits suicide every 100 minutes. Each year, approximately 1,900 adolescents take their own lives. According to the National Center for Health Statistics, in the United States, suicide is the fourth leading cause of adolescent death for teens between the ages of 10 and 13 and the third leading cause of death for teens between the ages of 15 and 19.

When discussing suicide, experts distinguish among suicidal ideation, suicide attempts, and completed suicides. Suicidal ideation refers to whether or not an individual has considered taking his or her own life and the nature and completeness of such thoughts. While many individuals may occasionally have fleeting thoughts of ending it all or wonder, for a brief moment, if life is worth continuing, most adolescents and adults do not move beyond such isolated thoughts. Yet, for others, these thoughts reoccur, and, in some cases, a person may begin to develop a plan about the circumstances and method that he or she would use to take his or her own life. There are also those labeled "attempters," people who indicate that they have actually attempted suicide.

According to the National Center for Injury Prevention and Control, in 2006, 17 percent of high school students attempted killing themselves in the previous year. Other researchers also found that 15 percent of high school students had developed a specific plan for carrying out a suicide. While females in the United States are more likely to think of suicide, to plan a suicide, and to attempt a suicide, males are more likely to complete a suicide. In fact, males in the United States are four times more likely to succeed in killing themselves than females.

Suicide rates also differ among groups of people. For example, the highest overall rates of adolescent suicide have been observed among Native Americans, followed by whites, and, in general, suicide has been less prevalent among African-American and Hispanic adolescents.

CONTRIBUTING FACTORS

Biology, family history, and a teen's personal characteristics contribute to suicidal ideation. Chemical and hormonal imbalances can leave an adolescent vulnerable to developing a mood disorder, such as depression. Also, suicidal behavior appears to run in families. Teens with a family history of suicide are more likely to complete suicide than those with no family history. Additionally, poor parent-child relationships have been linked to suicidal ideation. Teen suicide victims generally have been found to have less contact and less satisfying relationships with their parents compared to other teens.

The most salient factor related to adolescent suicide has been found to be the mental health of the teen. Research indicates that teen suicide is strongly related to previous suicide attempts, depression, bipolar disorder, substance abuse, problem gambling, and conduct disorder.

Inability to deal with normal life

Feeling down is a normal reaction to negative experiences that result in sadness, disappointment, and rejection. When teens suffer setbacks or frustrations in meeting challenges—failing an important exam, being rejected for admittance into the college of one's choice, the disintegration of a first love—they may feel depressed. Typically, however, these feelings of disappointment and sadness last only a limited period of time and diminish relatively quickly.

Yet, when sad feelings persist and begin to affect one's ability to function normally, then a serious condition called depression may develop. Depression is characterized by a wide range of feelings that may include dejection, guilt, hopelessness, and low self-esteem or a sense of worthlessness. Depression may also be accompanied by an inability to concentrate, a loss of or an increase in appetite, insomnia or sleeping too much, withdrawal from family and friends, and a lack of interest in favorite activities. For some, the symptoms associated with depression may feel so overwhelming that they may contemplate or even attempt suicide.

Call for help?

Certainly, suicidal ideation and suicide attempts are very serious matters; however, for many individuals, these thoughts and behaviors do not necessarily indicate a desire to die. For some, a suicide attempt may represent a dramatic call for help. For others, it may represent the wish to stop the psychic pain associated with disappointment or hopelessness.

ALTERNATIVE SOLUTIONS

While certain situations and their resultant feelings can generate significant psychological pain, individuals who contemplate suicide or act on suicidal thoughts often fail to consider three very important factors. First, there is almost always a solution to every problem. While at first glance, a situation or a problem may appear to be overwhelming, problems can be solved, and individuals who work through their problems usually experience a renewed sense of hope and an increased sense of self-confidence.

A second factor is the power of time. While strong, painful feelings may seem permanent to individuals contemplating suicide, heartache of the moment is not endless. Time itself is a great healer, a precious resource.

Human resiliency is the third factor usually overlooked by individuals contemplating suicide. The human spirit is remarkably and powerfully resilient. Even when confronted with a terrible tragedy like the untimely death of a loved one or the loss of one's home and savings, the human spirit, almost spontaneously, begins the process of healing and gradually, during this healing process, hope is eventually restored.

POOR COPING SKILLS

It is not uncommon to feel elevated stress levels in the face of adversity. However, coping skills and stress levels are related. Generally, the fewer the number of healthy coping skills, the more stress an individual experiences. Conversely, the greater the number of healthy coping skills, the less stress an individual feels.

The desire to avoid or escape one's problems is usually heightened among individuals who have underdeveloped or an insufficient number of coping skills. These individuals tend to develop maladaptive or poor coping skills, examples of which are using alcohol or drugs or engaging in other addictive activities, such as gambling, in order to deal with daily problems.

While alcohol, drugs, or gambling may provide a temporary sense of relief from uncomfortable feelings, these substances and activities do nothing to solve or resolve a person's preexisting problems (for example, parental, familial, academic, legal, vocational, peer, or personal stressors) that generate the feelings. In fact, rather than produce solutions, engaging in a maladaptive behavior to solve a problem actually creates more problems, exacerbates feelings of helplessness and hopelessness, and, in general, leaves an individual feeling even more overwhelmed or stressed-out than he or she was before taking a drink, using a drug, or placing a bet.

Coping skills and gambling

According to recent research, adolescents who meet the criteria for pathological gambling demonstrate poorer coping skills when compared to peers who do not have a gambling problem. When compared with non-gambling adolescents, adolescent problem gamblers demonstrate a reduced ability to successfully cope with stressful daily events, adversity, and situational problems; experience higher rates of depression and lower senses of self-esteem; and run a greater risk of developing another addiction or multiple addictions.

The most frequently cited, underlying, stress-producing problems reported by adolescent problem gamblers are personal (for example, low self-esteem, depression, ADHD), family conflict, issues with peers, and academic, legal, and vocational concerns. Also, adolescent problem gamblers report beginning gambling at earlier ages (approximately 10 years of age) as compared with peers without gambling problems. Additionally, the progression from social gambling to problem gambling is much more rapid for adolescents than for adults, and the prevalence rates for adolescent problem gambling are two to four times higher than they are for adults. Moreover, adolescents between the ages of 14 to 17 who have developed a gambling disorder are at an increased risk for suicidal ideation and suicide attempts.

THE LINK BETWEEN SUICIDE AND GAMBLING

Suicide represents a significant concern for individuals with gambling problems. According to the National Council on Problem Gambling, nearly 20 percent of pathological gamblers have attempted suicide. This figure is higher than the suicide rate for any other addictive disorder.

There are different views about the link between disordered gambling and suicide. Some experts suggest that the negative consequences and losses associated with gambling problems act as precipitants to the development of mood disorders, substance use disorders, and/or suicidal ideation and behaviors. However, other experts propose that preexisting problems, including mood disorders and/or substance abuse, both of which are highly associated with elevated risks for suicidal ideation or suicide attempts, are exacerbated by gambling problems and that the result of these additional gambling-related stresses increases a person's risk for suicide. Nonetheless, regardless of the order of onset or the cause,

DID YOU KNOW?

ADHD and Problem Gambling

According to a study of 462 children aged 7–11 with attention-deficit/hyperactivity disorder (ADHD) and a follow-up study when participants were 18 to 24 years old, young people with persistent ADHD ("persisters") have a higher rate (19.1%) of problem and pathological gambling (as compared to social or no gambling) than those young adults who have learned to cope with their symptoms of ADHD ("desisters").

Source: Adapted from Breyer, J. L., A. M. Botzet, K. C. Winters, R. D. Stinchfield, G. August, and G. Realmuto. "Young Adult Gambling Behaviors and Their Relationship with the Persistence of ADHD," *Journal of Gambling Studies*, 2009.

experts agree and clinical observations demonstrate that the rates of suicidal ideation and suicide attempts are elevated in problem and pathological gamblers compared with the general population.

WARNING SIGNS

The following points represent some general warning signs for both depression and suicidal ideation:

- talking about suicide, death, or "going away"
- talking about feelings of guilt or hopelessness
- giving away possessions and referring to things that "won't be needed"
- losing interest in favorite activities, such as being with friends and family
- having trouble concentrating
- exhibiting changes in eating and sleeping habits
- engaging in excessive gambling or alcohol and/or drug use

If you are concerned that you or someone you know are displaying these warning signs, contact the National Suicide Prevention Hotline at 1-800-SUICIDE (1-800-784-2433) or the National Suicide Prevention Lifeline at 1-800-273-TALK (1-800-273-8255).

See also: Addiction and Gambling; Adolescents and Gambling; Alcohol, Drugs, and Gambling; Depression and Pathological Gambling; Prevention and Intervention; Protective Factors

FURTHER READING

Feigelman, W., B. Gorman, and H. Lesieur. "Examining the Relationship Between At-risk Gambling and Suicidality in a National Representative Sample of Young Adults." *Suicide and Life-Threatening Behavior* 36 (2006).

Haley, James, ed. *Death & Dying* (Opposing Viewpoints Series). Farmington Hills, Mich.: Greenhaven Press, 2002.

Johnson, P., and M. Malow-Iroff. *Adolescents and Risk: Making Sense of Adolescent Psychology.* Westport, Conn.: Praeger Publishers, 2008.

Lezine, De Quincy, and David Brent. *Eight Stories Up: An Adolescent Chooses Hope over Suicide.* New York: Oxford University Press, 2008.

■ TYPES OF GAMBLING

Wagering on a multitude of games and activities. People can gamble on most every activity in which two or more outcomes are possible.

The most commonly thought of games consist of those found in a casino, table games, and slot machines. People also place wagers on sports events, horse racing, and lotteries. Although most people do not think of trading stocks on Wall Street as a form of gambling, the stock market is in fact a high-risk form of wagering.

Although gambling is legal in most of the world, there are many forms of illegal gambling, including underage gambling. Illegal forms of gambling consist of cockfighting, dogfighting, and gambling with a bookie.

TABLE GAMES

Poker is the most popular table game played in and outside of casinos. The games gleek, cribbage, lanterloo, bragg, and piquet have contributed to modern-day poker. Poker was first documented in Germany as the game *Pochen*, then migrated to France and became *poque*. The French introduced the game to the United States in New Orleans in the early 19th century. Poker became an instant hit on the Louisiana riverboats. The first poker game was played with 20 cards; the 52-card deck and the concept of the draw were developed around 1840. Since then, poker has developed into several styles, among them Omaha, Texas Hold 'Em, and seven- and five-card stud.

Blackjack is the second most played table game that consists of cards. Each player is dealt two cards; one card faces down, one up. The goal of the game is to beat the **dealer** and other players in attaining "21" with as few cards as possible.

Other table games consist of games that use dice or tiles. The most popular games in this category are craps, a dice game, and Pai Gow, a game that uses tiles. Craps is the descendant of Hazard, an English game that began as early as the Crusades. Hazard became the French crabs, which was brought to the United States through Louisiana and became craps. The most common craps game is played with one or more players against the **bank** or casino. The players place their bets on areas of the table that correspond to the outcome of two rolled dice. The game itself is complex and complicated. Pai Gow is a Chinese table game that uses tiles. Each player is dealt four tiles and separates the hand into high and low combinations. The players win if their hands beat the dealer's hand.

Roulette is a game of pure chance. It originated in France in the early 1700s, and by 1796, it evolved to be the game found in modern casinos. The goal of the game is to bet on either colors or numbers in a wheel with slots, spin the wheel, and hope the outcome is in the player's favor.

Bingo and keno are also common games of chance found in casinos or locations where gambling is legal. Bingo is played with a sheet of numbers, the goal being to fill up a horizontal, diagonal, or vertical line with randomly called numbers. Once a player has completed the line, he or she calls bingo and collects the winnings. Keno is a Chinese game similar to bingo in that it relies on randomly selected numbers. The players in keno select their numbers before the round and win if their numbers are called.

SLOT MACHINES AND VIDEO POKER

Slot machines originated around 1899, when Charles Fey invented the first nickel-accepting "Liberty Bell." The Liberty Bell was a reel machine where the right combination of symbols paid out a sum of money. A combination of three bells paid the highest sum. The other symbols most commonly found on the machine were card suits and horseshoes. Although Charles Fey invented the first slot machine, Herbert Mills, a Chicago-based manufacturer, made the machines popular through mass production. Most of the early slot machines did not pay in monetary compensation; instead, they dispensed novelties like candy, cigars, and tokens for extra play. Slot machines gained immediate popularity, as they gave consumers an entertaining way to spend their time and maybe even win a cigar or two. Slot machines became an instant hit and are found in all casinos worldwide.

Video poker machines are similar to slot machines, although winning on them does not rely purely on chance. These machines were invented in the 1880s and allowed patrons to play poker in solitude. As technology advanced, so did the poker machines. Today, video poker stations are mostly touch-screen games.

SPORTS BETTING AND HORSE RACING

Sports betting can be traced back to ancient Rome where wagering on chariot races was popular. Sports betting in America was brought over from England where pedestrianism, a game of competitive walking, was a popular sport. Pedestrianism lost popularity with the dawn of competitive sports like baseball. Bets can be made on most every aspect of every sport ranging from the outcome of the game to how many points each team has at different parts of the game.

Horse racing is another sport that has been around since ancient Rome. The English brought horse racing to colonial America in the mid-1600s. Although legal today, wagering on horse races was banned in almost every state during the early 1900s. There are three types of horse racing—thoroughbred, quarter horse, and endurance races. Thoroughbred racing is the most widely known type of racing. The Kentucky Derby, the Preakness, and the Belmont Stakes—a series of races known as the Triple Crown—are all thoroughbred events. This type of racing occurs on an oval track and is based on the speed and endurance of the horse. Quarter horse racing takes place on a mile-long straight track with quarter horses. Endurance races take place on long trails and can last for days, varying from 10 to 100 miles.

THE STOCK EXCHANGE

Trading stocks can be traced back to 12th-century France. Buying stock in a company is a form of wagering because it is high risk and the outcome is variable. A person might buy stock in a little-known company at a low price. If that company succeeds, the buyer's compensation rises with the growth of the company. If the company loses money or closes down, the buyer loses money. Many people watch the stock market and attempt to buy and sell based on economic predictions. The stock market moves quickly and can be unpredictable, which results in an intense and adrenaline-filled atmosphere.

ILLEGAL GAMBLING

Gambling is not legal in every country or state; therefore, any type of gambling that is prohibited, including underage gambling, is illegal. However, even in countries where some forms of gambling are legal, the most harmful types of gambling are illegal. Cockfighting and dogfighting are two of the most infamous examples of illegal gambling.

Cockfighting began in Southeast Asia and spread like wildfire through Europe and then America. The roosters used for cockfighting are bred to kill. They are sometimes dressed in artificial spurs to aid the process. Patrons wager on which rooster comes out alive.

Although cockfighting has been banned in all 50 U.S. states, due especially to cruelty, underground games still exist.

Dogfighting was brought to the United States from England and Ireland in the 1830s. American pit bull terriers are the dogs most commonly bred to fight. Dogfighting is a brutal and deadly sport. The dogs are trained to kill by using smaller animals as bait, starvation, and violence. The more abused a dog is, the deadlier he will be in the pit. If the losing dog is not killed in the pit, he is often discarded or executed for entertainment. The sport was outlawed in the 1860s but is still widespread throughout America.

Gambling is not limited to casino games, sports betting, or the various types of illegal gambling activities. Wagers can be placed on any activity that has multiple outcomes. Although the games can be entertaining, most are high risk and do not have favorable outcomes, with the obvious chance of losing and the ever present house advantage.

Q & A

Question: What is the house advantage?

Answer: The house advantage is the percentage that a casino expects to make on a wager. All casino games are designed to have a house advantage; it is how they make money from slot machines and table games. Most house-advantage percentages for both table and slot games range from as little as 0.5 percent to as much as 17 percent. In short, eventually the casino always wins, making gambling a risky activity.

FURTHER READING

Durham, S., and K. Hashimoto. *The History of Gambling in America: Balancing Costs and Benefits of Legalized Gambling.* Upper Saddle River, N.J.: Pearson Education, 2010.

Schwartz, David G. *Roll the Bones: The History of Gambling.* New York: Gotham Books, 2006.

▪ UNDERAGE GAMBLING

See: Adolescents and Gambling; Law and Gambling, The

■ VIDEO GAME PLAYING

Video and computer games are an increasingly large part of adolescent life. A study conducted by the Pew Internet and American Life Project found that 99 percent of adolescent boys and 94 percent of adolescent girls play video games regularly. Researchers also have found that video games and gambling are similar and that playing video games may lead to future problems with gambling.

VIDEO GAMES AND PROBLEM GAMBLING

Problem gamblers are more likely to spend excessive amounts of time playing video or computer games. Some experts believe that playing video or computer games also may lead to the development of problem gambling in teens and that this may occur because video games are similar in style to video lottery terminals, which are automated gambling machines such as slot machines, video poker and blackjack machines, and keno.

Adolescents may begin gambling for the same reasons they play video games. In other words, many people use gaming or gambling to escape or disassociate from their problems or negative emotions. The stimulation may increase mood or relieve tension and stress. Evading problems in this way can lead to excessive gaming.

Both video games and video lottery terminals award points when a gamer completes a task. This type of point system positively reinforces the game-playing behavior. Some online games take the point system to a whole new level. Players can actually purchase points to play games, letting them move through the game more easily.

Video lottery terminals work in the same way as some video games. The player pays for his or her credits or points. In both situations, playing for the longest amount of time on the least amount of points or credits is considered a success. Arcade games are video games, too. They require payment before each play. Sometimes tickets are issued if the player does well. The tickets can be turned in for a prize. This system is like that of slot machines in a casino, where a gambler is issued a ticket that can be turned in for cash. The similarities between point systems make transforming from a gamer to a gambler all too easy.

Reinforcers and rewards

Video games have the same visual and auditory reinforcers as automated gambling such as slot machines and roulette. **Reinforcement** is a term used in the psychological theory of "operant conditioning." When an individual is given a prize or praise for completing a behavior, the prize or praise acts as a reinforcer, which causes the individual to increase that behavior. With both video games and gambling machines, when a player does something well, sounds and pictures flash to act as a reinforcer for repeating this activity.

Game playing and gambling have the same type of reward schedule. Being rewarded while playing video games is based on skill level: the better the player, the more levels he or she is able to complete or the more points he or she accrues. Many assume they can gain mastery over gambling in the same ways they can develop skill in video game playing. However, this is not the case: Success in gambling using video lottery terminals is based purely on chance.

THE INFLUENCE OF PEERS

Peer relationships are important during adolescence. They help adolescents develop healthy relationships and act as a normal outlet to cope with family stress. Research has shown that healthy peer relationships can lead to higher self-esteem and academic success. Peer relationships can also be negative. Teens often seek approval through friends, and friendship can result in competition, healthy or otherwise. Because video games are often played in groups—either in person or online—young people can get caught up in excessive game playing as a way to fit in. In turn, individuals may begin gambling as a result of peer pressure, allowing the need to fit in to outweigh the decision to refrain from risky activities.

Boys versus girls

Experts believe that male video gamers are more susceptible to developing problems with gambling. Males tend to spend more time per week gambling than females who are the same age. Boys polled in a recent research study found playing video games to be exciting, relaxing, and a way to lose track of time with friends. The same study found that female adolescents played video games at substantially lesser rates. The reasons for this may be that females are not socialized to play video games and that boys are given more opportunities to play video games. In fact, video games are usually marketed for male users. Interestingly, the games marketed for female users are usually unlike games found on video lottery terminals; instead, they are games using trivia, cooking, and taking care of pets or children.

Another reason for the gender difference in playing video games is that males tend to have stronger visual and spatial skills than females, while females are typically stronger in languages. Consequently, males will be more drawn to and succeed more often in playing video games.

The results

Because playing video games is considered a male-dominated activity, females are rarely rewarded for participating and in fact may be ostracized for taking part. Due to this heavy male presence in video game playing, males are more susceptible to developing a gambling problem. However, female players are not exempt. Female gamers who play video games excessively develop gambling problems at the same rate as their male counterparts.

Q & A

Question: Can playing video games cause teens to be violent or result in physical injury? Can it also lead to a gambling problem?

Answer: Many studies show that adolescents who play violent games exhibit an increase in aggressiveness, although most studies did not show long-term effects. There are also numerous physical effects of excessive video game playing, such as changes in blood pressure and heart rate, eye strain, and repetitive strain injury. The latter is the most common ailment caused by prolonged video game playing. It is a result of holding or consistently moving a part of one's body in the same position for extended amounts of time. For example, operating a video game controller for a prolonged period of time may cause repetitive strain injury on the wrists, fingers, and elbows. Also, although not all adolescents who play video games will develop a gambling problem, there is a clear link between the two activities.

CONCLUSIONS

Video game playing clearly can lead to problems with gambling. The similarities between the two activities are extensive. Also, in recent years, online gambling has blurred the line between game playing and gambling. As of 2009 in the United States, 87 percent of young people, ages 12 to 17, were Internet users. Also, despite its illegal status, 300,000 young adults, ages 14–21, gamble online weekly, and 700,000 young people gamble online at least monthly, according to another 2009 study. Because online gambling is more easily accessible to adolescents now than ever before, the risk of adolescents' developing gambling problems is heightened.

See also: Family Life and Gambling; Internet and Online Gambling, The; Peer Pressure and Gambling; Youth at Special Risk

FURTHER READING
Johnson, P., and M. Malow-Iroff. *Adolescents and Risk: Making Sense of Adolescent Psychology.* Santa Barbara, Calif.: Praeger Publishers, 2008.

■ YOUTH AT SPECIAL RISK

Adolescents with increased chances of becoming problem gamblers. Studies show that the rates among adolescents of problem gambling (3.5 to 8 percent) and of at-risk gambling (10 to 15 percent) are higher than the rates found among adults. Estimates show that 85 percent of high school students have gambled in their lifetimes, and approximately 73 percent of that 85 percent had gambled within the past 12 months. Also, 4 to 7 percent of adolescents appear to meet the diagnostic criteria for pathological gambling and are classified as "problem" gamblers.

Due to their developmental stage—a time of change, growth, and exploration—adolescents are prone to risk-taking behaviors, and gambling is a risky activity. It appeals to the adolescent population because of the chance to win, spend time with friends, or just get away from problems for a while. Typically, from a young age, children and teens are exposed to gambling activities such as school raffles, fundraisers, bingo, and other contests found in schools, making gambling seem commonplace.

BOYS VERSUS GIRLS

Estimates indicate that the ratio of boys to girls with severe gambling-related problems is in the range of 3:1 to 5:1. In examining other gender differences, adult female pathological gamblers are reported to generally start gambling at a later age than men, with their gambling problems developing more rapidly. In contrast, adult male pathological gamblers exhibit more problems with impulse control. Research also shows that males prefer games of strategy (for example, poker or sports betting), while females are more likely to participate in non-strategic games (for example, slot machines or bingo). Overall, male problem gamblers tend to be more competitive and concerned with winning and losing, while females are more likely to become problem gamblers out of a need to escape problems.

STUDENT ATHLETES

Student athletes are among the young people at special risk for problem gambling. Approximately two-thirds of college athletes gamble, specifically, one-third of collegiate male athletes and 10 percent of female athletes bet on college sports in the last year. Division III college athletes, those in smaller schools, are the most likely to gamble. Also, because athletes often tend to be risk takers and are competitive, they are perhaps predisposed to gambling. The thrill of competition and the drive to win make sports a potential breeding ground for the development of risk-taking behaviors.

Fact Or Fiction?

Boys gamble more than girls.

The Facts: Studies have found that males gamble more than females. Males spend more time playing video games, sports, and cards, and each of these activities has a gambling component. Also, video game playing often translates into online gambling.

As adolescents grow accustomed to these games, they feel the need to up the ante and find an activity with a higher risk potential. Gambling has this high-risk potential. Watching and playing sports also can result in gambling, and seeing parents bet on sports like football can influence children and teens to mimic that behavior. Females, on the other hand, tend to be socialized to participate in other types of activities, although some do gamble.

MINORITIES AND GAMBLING

Like student athletes, young members of certain minority groups are more likely to gamble and exhibit gambling-related problems.

Researchers have observed adolescent problem gamblers to be more prevalent among minority ethnic groups, including Hispanics. Studies have found that approximately 10 percent of African-American, American-Indian, and Mexican-American youth gamble daily, compared to only 4 percent of Caucasian and 5 percent of Asian-American youth.

Native Americans

Research has shown that Native American teenagers gamble at younger ages and are more likely to experience gambling-related problems, earlier onset of problems from gambling, and greater frequency of such problems than were their non-Native American peers. According to the South Oaks Gambling Screen, 9.6 percent of a sample group of Native American teens met the criteria for pathological gambling, a prevalence rate that was significantly higher than the 5.6 percent reported for non-native adolescents. In the same study, Native Americans were also found to gamble more frequently and start at an earlier age. Additionally, perhaps because of a cultural stigma or a lack of available treatment, they are often less likely to seek professional help, leaving the untreated problem gambler at risk for having more problems.

African Americans

Recent studies indicate that nearly one-quarter of African-American adolescents are at-risk gamblers and 13 percent are problem gamblers. African Americans living in disadvantaged neighborhoods had much higher rates of problem and pathological gambling as compared to those who did not live in disadvantaged neighborhoods. Although research shows that African Americans in general gamble less frequently than Hispanics and Caucasians, they have larger numbers of heavy gamblers. Also, according to researchers at The Institute for Gambling Education and Research at the University of Memphis, "African American young men who have a parent who gambles are more likely to gamble frequently and to perceive themselves as having gambling problems." Additionally, "young African American men in families with no set rules in the home . . . were more likely to be identified as problem gamblers," suggesting that family functioning is very important in influencing gambling involvement by this group.

Hispanic Americans

Studies show that 10 percent of Mexican-American youth gamble on a daily basis compared to 4 percent of their Caucasian counterparts. Research indicates that acculturation difficulties, economic hardships, and lower levels of education may play a role in the creation of pathological gambling. Hispanic and African-American males are also less likely to seek professional help for any issues they may face.

Fact Or Fiction?

African-American and Hispanic men and boys who are problem gamblers don't like to seek professional help.

The Facts: African-American and Hispanic males are less likely to get help for gambling problems. This may be a result of accessibility to help or the stigma attached to seeking mental health counseling of any kind.

Lack of accessibility to mental health services can stem from low income, remote location, and difficulty finding and affording child care. In addition, some insurance companies do not include mental health services in their policies, and those that do often fail to provide coverage for pathological gambling. Without insurance coverage, the costs of counseling and rehabilitation of gambling problems can be high.

Locating a mental health clinic that offers problem gambling support also can be difficult, and the distance may be too far to travel easily by bus or car. For single fathers or fathers whose spouse also works, affording both counseling and a babysitter may pose another problem.

Finally, for many African-American and Hispanic males, there is a stigma associated with counseling, which can be seen as a "feminine" activity. These men do not seek out services because they may feel it compromises their masculinity.

CULTURE

People's culture or environment influences their behavior. For example, cultures that approve of or endorse gambling tend to have higher rates of pathological gambling. Also, gambling has become a socially accepted form of entertainment and is often romanticized in popular culture. Finally, research has shown that higher rates of problem and pathological gambling exist in adolescents whose parents gamble.

YOUTH IN DETENTION

Adolescents in juvenile detention facilities are another group at an increased risk for gambling problems. Pathological gambling rates among incarcerated teens range from 18 to 38 percent. Studies also show that 42.4 percent of adolescents with gambling problems have borrowed or stolen money; 21 percent have committed illegal acts; 24 percent stole money from their family; and 23 percent stole from outside the family to cover gambling debts or to continue gambling. One study indicated that 18 percent of incarcerated youth met the criteria for problem gambling, and 54.5 percent of that group had gambled in the last week.

See also: Adolescents and Gambling; Crime and Gambling; Family Life and Gambling; Gender and Gambling; Sports and Gambling

FURTHER READING
Lancelot, M. *Gripped by Gambling.* Tucson, Ariz.: Wheatmark, 2007.
Lee, B. *Born to Lose.* Center City, Minn.: Hazelden Press, 2005.

HOTLINES AND HELP SITES

Gam-Anon
URL: http://www.gam-anon.org/
Phone: 1-718-352-1671
Fax: 1-718-746-2571
Address: P.O. Box 157
Whitestone, NY 11357
Mission: To help the family and friends of compulsive gamblers understand the problem of gambling and learn appropriate methods of dealing with the gambler
Programs: Weekly meetings are open to those affected by the gambling problems of another.

Gamblers Anonymous
URL: http://www.gamblersanonymous.org/
Phone: 1-213-386-8789
Fax: 1-213-386-0030
Address: P.O. Box 17173
Los Angeles, CA 90017
Mission: To help gamblers break their addiction through mutual help and support
Program: This is a twelve-step treatment program for gambling addiction.

Institute for Research on Gambling Disorders
URL: www.gamblingdisorders.org

Phone: 1-978-299-3040
Fax: 1-978-524-4162
Address: 100 Cummings Center
Suite 207P
Beverly, MA 01970
Affiliation: National Center for Responsible Gaming (NCRG)
Mission: To manage and administer a competitive research grants program and conduct public awareness and education about gambling disorders; Web site offers a wide collection of resources about gambling disorders

Medline Plus
URL: http://www.nlm.nih.gov/medlineplus/compulsivegambling.html
Affiliation: National Institutes of Health (NIH)
Mission: Provides links to articles on treatment, studies, news, and other Web sites about gambling addiction

National Center for Responsible Gaming (NCRG)
URL: www.ncrg.org
Phone: 1-202-552-2689
Fax: 1-202-552-2676
Address: 1299 Pennsylvania Avenue, NW
Suite 1175
Washington, DC 20004
Mission: To help individuals and families affected by gambling disorders by supporting the finest peer-reviewed, scientific research into pathological and youth gambling; to encourage the application of new research findings to improve prevention, diagnostic, intervention, and treatment strategies; and to advance public education about responsible gaming and gambling disorders

National Council on Problem Gambling
URL: http://www.ncpgambling.org/
Phone: 1-202-547-9204
Fax: 1-202-547-9206
Address: 730 11th Street, NW
Suite 601
Washington, DC 20001
Mission: To increase public awareness of pathological gambling, ensure the widespread availability of treatment for problem gamblers and

their families, and to encourage research and programs for prevention and education

National Hotline for Problem Gambling
Phone: 1-800-522-4700 (24-hour confidential national hotline)
Affiliation: National Council on Problem Gambling
Mission: To provide a 24-hour confidential national hotline for people who are affected by problem gambling

GLOSSARY

abstinence   the practice of not engaging in a behavior, such as sexual relations, drinking, or gambling

abuse   the misuse of a substance or mistreatment of a person, causing injury

addictive   causing a psychological, emotional, or physical need for a substance such as alcohol, tobacco, or drugs, or for an activity, such as gambling

addicts   people with a psychological, emotional, or physical need for a substance or behavior such as alcohol, tobacco, drugs, or gambling

ADHD (attention-deficit/hyperactivity disorder)   the most common neurobiological and behavioral disorder in children, symptoms of which include distractibility, impulsivity, and hyperactivity

adolescence   the stage of growth and development between childhood and adulthood entailing major physical, cognitive, emotional, and social changes

adrenaline   a hormone secreted in the adrenal gland and produced in response to fear

Alcoholics Anonymous (AA) the first and largest self-help group for alcoholics

alcoholism a physical and psychological dependence on alcohol

anxiety abnormal sense of fear, doubt about reality of the source of the fear, and self-doubt about coping with it

bank the fund of supplies (as money, chips, or pieces) held by the banker or dealer for use in gaming

bipolar disorder a brain disorder that causes extreme shifts in a person's energy, mood, and ability to function; also known as manic-depressive illness

bookie short for "bookmaker," one who determines odds and receives and pays off bets

casino a building or room used for gambling

chemical a substance that is manufactured through chemistry; in terms of drug use, a product that does not occur naturally in the environment

chronic long-lasting or repeated; used to describe any persistent behavior or illness, such as **alcoholism,** that is not easily cured

cognitive behavioral therapy (CBT) psychological therapy where patients work to understand the thoughts and emotions behind their behavior

comorbidity the presence of two or more disorders within a single individual

compulsion uncontrollable urge to do something

compulsive feeling uncontrollable urges to do something over and over; obsessive, repetitive, ritualized

conduct disorder a term used to describe a pattern of repetitive behavior where the rights of others or the current social norms are violated; symptoms often include verbal and physical aggression, cruel behavior toward people and animals, and other destructive behavior such as lying, stealing, truancy, and vandalism

dealer the person who operates table games such as dice, roulette, or cards in a casino

dependency an intense physical or psychological need for a behavior or a substance, such as alcohol, without which a dependent person suffers severe discomfort or illness

disorder *See* mental disorder

dissociative separating segments of the personality from the mainstream of consciousness or behavior

dopamine a brain chemical, classified as a neurotransmitter, found in regions of the brain that regulate movement, emotion, motivation, and pleasure

dopaminergic dysfunction a failure of the neural pathways involved with dopamine transmission

gaming another term for gambling

gateway (drug or behavior) the first drug, often alcohol, used by people who later use illegal drugs or engage in illegal activity

genetic relating to an inherited or familial trait or disease

group therapy treatment in which a group of people meet with mental health professionals to talk with each other about how to deal with and resolve problems

house advantage in games of chance, the superior position that a casino holds over a player; also, the percentage that a casino expects to make from a wager

impulse control the ability to control one's behavior in a specific situation

impulse-control disorder mental disorder that is characterized by an individual's inability to remain in control of his or her behavior

impulsive acting before thinking the situation through

interest rates rates which are charged a borrower for the use of money

interventions skilled techniques and activities that make up a treatment plan, particularly for a problem behavior

lotteries games, often state-run, in which people play numbers of their choice in a random drawing

mental disorder a clinically significant psychological or psychiatric condition

money laundering hiding the source of illegal funds by means of legitimate business channels

neurobiological of or relating to an illness of the nervous system caused by genetic, metabolic, or other biological factors

neurotransmitter a neurochemical, such as **serotonin,** that attaches to a receptor in the brain to transfer signals between a neuron and another cell

noradrenergic dysfunction a dysregulation of the neurotransmitter norepinephrine, a dysfunction often implicated with depression

obsessive-compulsive disorder a form of anxiety characterized by recurring and intrusive thoughts, feelings, or ideas (obsessions) and/or the need to repeat certain patterns of behavior (compulsions)

panic attack an episode of extreme anxiety; the recurring crisis phase of a panic disorder

pathological   due to or related to a disease

peer   an individual of one's own age and/or economic or social status

point spread   a specified number of points by which it is wagered that a sports team must win or lose

progressive disorder   a condition, such as alcohol abuse, that tends to get worse with time

puberty   the time of life when the sex glands begin to function

rehabilitation   process of restoring to a former condition of health

reinforcement   giving an individual a prize or praise for completing a behavior, which causes the individual to increase that behavior

remission   state of health after a medicine or therapy has destroyed a disease or treated a problem

risk   any action for which there is some possibility of failure as well as some opportunity for success

risk factor   anything, such as family background or personal problems, that might put a person at high risk for alcohol abuse, developing a gambling problem, or other dangerous outcomes

science of probability   a mathematical theory of whether or not an event will occur at random

self-esteem   the sense of value one attributes to oneself; one's opinion of oneself

serotonergic dysfunction   a failure of the neural pathways involved with serotonin transmission

serotonin   a neurotransmitter or chemical that inhibits self-destructive behavior; also affects a person's mood and feelings of being hungry or full

shaving points   illegally promising money to an athlete who ensures his or her team will either lose or not cover the point spread

socioeconomic status   an economic measure based on an individual's or family's income, occupation, and education

stigma   a socially unacceptable characteristic or behavior that causes a person shame or to be looked down upon

stimulant   a drug, such as caffeine, nicotine, amphetamine, or cocaine, that tends to temporarily increase alertness, energy, and physical activity

stress   emotional strain or discomfort felt from the pressures of life

stressor   a factor or event that precipitates or drives a negative behavior or outcome

tolerance   a need to increase the size or frequency of bets/substance use

trigger   a factor or event that initiates and aggravates a specific behavior or a response

twelve-step program   any treatment program for alcoholism, problem gambling, or other addiction that stresses the Twelve Steps to recovery developed by **Alcoholics Anonymous**

underage   legally considered to be a child

wager   a bet, usually of money, on a game

withdrawal   the physical symptoms connected with ending the use of addictive drugs or addictive behaviors, such as problem gambling

INDEX

Boldface page numbers indicate extensive treatment of a topic.

A

Arizona Office of Problem Gambling 84
Arkansas, gambling age in 72
astragali 54
athletes 107–109, 127
Atlantic City, Georgia 64, 102
attention-deficit hyperactivity disorder 116
Augustus (emperor of Rome) 55
Australia 101
avoidance-focused skills 79

B

bailouts 45
Belmont Stakes 121
Bible 55
binge drinking 37
binge eating 37–38
binge gambling **36–40**
   biological factors 38–39
   defining the binge concept 36–38
   personality traits 39–40
bingo 120
biomedical model of addiction 12–13
bio-psycho-social model of addiction 13
bipolar disorder 70
blackjack 59, 119
Blaszczynski, A. 36
bookies 22, 109
bragg 119
brain, changes in 16, 34, 38
Business of Risk, The (Abt) 74

C

California, gambling age in 72
California gold rush 57
California v. Cabazon Band of Mission Indians 57
Caligula (emperor of Rome) 55
Canada 101
Canterbury Tales, The (Chaucer) 55
cards, playing 55–56
casinos 40, 56, 102
casual social gamblers 103–104
Catholic Church 56
CBT. *See* cognitive behavioral therapy
Central City Opera House Association, Chames v. 68
Chames v. Central City Opera House Association 68
characteristics of gamblers 4–6
"chasing the loss" 43, 109
Chaucer, Geoffrey 55

children, as victims 51–53
China 56
Claudius (emperor of Rome) 55
cocaine 32
cockfighting 121–122
codes of conduct 28
cognitive behavioral therapy 48–49, 63, 64
cognitive-behavior model of addiction 12
Colorado, gambling age in 72
commitment risks 95
comorbidity 31–34
compulsion 36
compulsive/pathological gamblers 104
computer games. *See* video game playing
conduct disorder 114
Connecticut, gambling age in 72
consequences of gambling
   familial 49–54
   and online gambling 69
   and public health issues 91
   and sports gambling 109
coping skills 79, 81, 114, 115–116
counseling. *See* help for gamblers
craps 59, 119
credit card debt 43–44, 69
cribbage 119
crime and gambling **40–45**. *See also* law and gambling
   adolescent gambling and 42–43
   debt and credit 43–45
   money problems and 43
   types of criminal activity 40–42
culture and gambling 129–130
Custer, Robert 102–103, 108

D

Dayshire studies 52
debt and credit 43–44
Delaware, gambling age in 72
Department of Justice 40, 68
depression **45–49**
   and adolescent gambling 79
   and alcohol/drugs 32
   and debt 45
   gambling and addiction 46
   symptoms of 46–48
   treatment of co-occurring disorders 48–49
Derevensky, Jeffrey L. 4–5
developmental assets 84